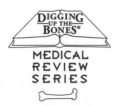

MEDICAL
REVIEW
SERIES

# Obstetrics
# and Gynecology

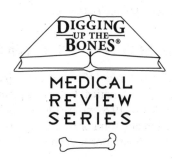

# Obstetrics and Gynecology

Compiled and Written by
**Sonia Lott, M.D.**

**Nikos M. Linardakis, M.D.**
Editor-in-Chief
Digging Up the Bones Series

**McGRAW-HILL**
Health Professions Division

New York  St. Louis  San Francisco  Auckland  Bogotá  Caracas  Lisbon  London
Madrid  Mexico City  Milan  Montreal  New Delhi  San Juan  Singapore  Sydney
Tokyo  Toronto

# McGraw-Hill

A Division of The McGraw-Hill Companies

**OBSTETRICS AND GYNECOLOGY: Digging Up the Bones**

1234567890 MALMAL 998

ISBN 0-07-038220-4

This book was set in Times Roman by V & M Graphics, Inc.
The editors were John Dolan and Steven Melvin;
the production supervisor was Helene G. Landers;
the cover designer was Matthew Dvorozniak;
the index was prepared by Jerry Ralya;
assistant editor was Mary Martin Cadieux, M.D.;
illustrations and graphic assistance by Eric Melander and
Nikos M. Linardakis, M.D.

Malloy Lithographing, Inc., was the printer and binder.

**Library of Congress Cataloging-in-Publication Data**

Linardakis, Nikos M.
   Obstetrics & gynecology / compiled and written by Nikos M.
Linardakis and Sonia Lott.
     p.   c.m. — (Digging up the bones)
    ISBN 0-07-038220-4
    1. Obstetrics—Outlines, syllabi, etc.    2. Gynecology—Outlines
syllabi, etc.    I. Lott, Sonia.    II. Title.    III. Series: Digging up
the bones medical review series.
    [DNLM: 1. Pregnancy. 2. Genital Diseases, Female. 3. Genitalia,
Female.    WQ 200 L735o    1998]
RG533.L56    1998
618—dc21
DNLM/DLC
for Library of Congress          98-10207

*In loving memory of Zella Lott, my mother, best friend, and guardian angel—S.L.*

*To Mrs. Sophia Petrakos, my lifetime family friend.—N.M.L.*

# Contents

# Preface

Prepare to pass your exams! *Digging Up the Bones* medical review series will supply you with a quick facts review of the highly tested material in medicine. This volume of *Digging Up the Bones* was written by Sonia Lott, M.D., a recent Obstetrics and Gynecology resident, and edited in collaboration with leading physician, Mary Martin Cadieux, M.D. We hope you enjoy this clear and expressive book as it covers the topics in Obstetrics and Gynecology rotations and examinations. This book will complement your current understanding and primary instructional books. We recommend reviewing *Obstetrics and Gynecology* at least two times to memorize and understand the material. Always think of clinically related scenarios to help in the learning process.

*Digging Up the Bones Obstetrics and Gynecology* presents incredible diagrams and illustrations (in collaboration with the graphic medical illustrator, Eric Melander) in an easy-to-review format. Take the time to understand all of the illustrations. Remember, "a picture is worth a thousand words." You will grasp the topics more clearly from studying each illustration. We also pinpoint essential clinical scenarios, focusing on key highlights and summarizing the material most likely to be seen on your exams. Take the time to read EVERYTHING in this book and become familiar with these details—they are likely to show up on your exams!

As with all books, please use this review book as a "tool" to do well on your exams. These high-yield clinical facts will be of tremendous help. As with all books in this series I would appreciate the feedback of both students and physicians for the continuing improvement of this book; my e-mail address is DrLinard@aol.com.

Now that you have the information available to you in a dramatic and concise format, I know you will be comfortable and knowledgeable with your exams.

Nikos M. Linardakis, M.D.

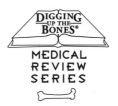

# Obstetrics
# and Gynecology

# Anatomy Overview 1

---

## *UTERUS*

### PARTS
**Fundus**: upper region of the uterus
**Cornu**: fallopian tubes enter here
**Corpus**: body
**Cervix**: the narrow, inferior part of the uterus
> *cervical canal* is approximately 2.5 cm long and
> separates the internal os and the external os
> *internal os* separates cervix from corpus
> *external os (opening of the canal)* separates cervix from vagina

### LAYERS OF CORPUS
**Mesometrium:** serosal layer that is the reflection of the visceral peritoneum
**Myometrium:** smooth muscle layer in three parts—outer longitudinal, middle oblique, and inner longitudinal
**Endometrium** (Fig. 1-1): columnar mucosal layer that undergoes cyclic changes during the menstrual cycle (see Chap. 6 for discussion).

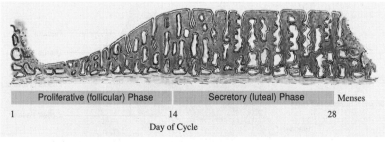

| Proliferative (follicular) Phase | Secretory (luteal) Phase | Menses |
|---|---|---|
| 1 | 14 | 28 |

Day of Cycle

**Figure 1-1** Normal endometrium, shown in varying phases of the menstrual cycle.

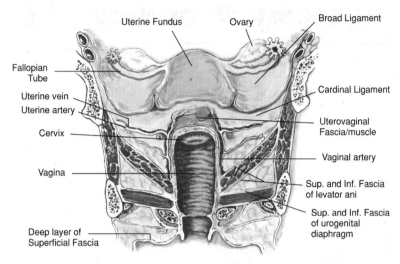

**Figure 1-2**    Supporting structures of the pelvic viscera

## LIGAMENTS (Fig. 1-2)

**Broad ligaments:** peritoneum that extends from lateral pelvic wall over uterus and adnexa

**Round ligaments:** fold of peritoneum that extends from the corpus downward and laterally between the two layers of the mesometrium toward the inguinal canal and terminates in the labia majora vestigial, which is the gubernaculum in the female (this ligament stretches during pregnancy)

**Cardinal ligaments** (Fig. 1-3): subserous fascia that extends from the uterus to the lateral pelvic wall and contains the uterine blood supply; provides support for middle and upper one-third of the cervix and vagina

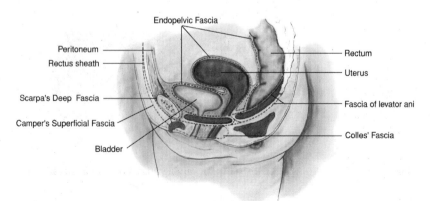

**Figure 1-3**    Fascia of the pelvis

**Uterosacral ligaments:** inferior posterior peritoneal folds from the broad ligament that extend from the sacrum around the rectum to the cervix

### BLOOD SUPPLY
**Uterine arteries:** vessels arise from each internal iliac artery. Branches of the uterine artery are the ascending and descending (vaginal) branches. The uterine artery will become hypertrophic during pregnancy (to provide adequate blood flow to the uterus and placenta).
**Ovarian arteries:** anastomoses with the uterines in the mesometrium

### NERVE SUPPLY
Superior hypogastric plexus
Inferior hypogastric plexus
Common iliac nerves: arise separately from the superior hypogastric plexus
Visceral afferents from the uterus: pain is referred to the **S2–S4** dermatomes
1. Nervi erigentes: sensory components, visceral afferents from the cervical region
2. Afferents from the body of the uterus and the tubes are parallel to the sympathetic pathway. Pain is referred to the **T12–L2** dermatomes (occurs with salpingitis).

---

## FALLOPIAN TUBES (OVIDUCTS)
The fallopian tubes run from the superior uterine angles through the superior border of the broad ligaments to the region of the ovaries.

### PARTS
Isthmus
Ampulla
Infundibulum: fimbriae are at end

### LAYERS
Serous: peritoneum
Subserous or adventitial: vascular and fibrous; blood and nerve supply
Muscular: outer longitudinal and inner circular
Mucosa

### LIGAMENTS
Infundibulopelvic ligament

### BLOOD SUPPLY
Derived from the ovarian and uterine arteries.

### NERVE SUPPLY
Pelvic plexuses for parasympathetic and sympathetic
Ovarian plexus

## VAGINA

Extends from the uterus to the vestibule of the external genitalia and opens to the outside. The fornix is the circular cul-de-sac around the cervix consisting of four regions: two lateral regions, one anterior and one posterior region. It pierces the urogenital diaphragm at its inferior end and is surrounded by two bulbocavernous muscles that act as sphincters. The hymen is an incomplete fold of highly vascularized tissue and mucous membrane, present in the virginal state, which partially separates the vaginal opening (the hymen covers the inferior portion of the vaginal lumen). During the first coitus, the hymen is usually stretched (and torn).

### SUPPORTS
The bulbocavernous muscles support it at the introitus.
The levator ani (puborectalis) muscles at the lower one-third.
Lower one-third includes the pelvic diaphragm, urogenital diaphragm, and the perineal body.
Middle one-third includes the pelvic diaphragm and the cardinal ligament.
Upper one-third includes the cardinal ligament and the uterosacral ligament.

### LAYERS
Mucosa is made up of stratified squamous epithelium.
Smooth muscle consists of an outer longitudinal layer, a circumferential layer that envelops the urethra in the lower one-third, and an inner longitudinal layer.

### BLOOD SUPPLY
Chief supply through the vaginal branch of the uterine artery.
The hypogastric artery gives blood supply through the middle rectal artery and the inferior vaginal artery.

### NERVE SUPPLY
The hypogastric plexus supplies the sympathetic innervation.
The pelvic nerve supplies the parasympathetic innervation.

## PELVIC MUSCULATURE

**Psoas major** flexes the spine and pelvis and abducts the lumbar region.
The **iliacus** along with the psoas makes up the most powerful thigh flexor and acts as a lateral rotator of the femur with the foot off the ground and frees and acts as a medial rotator with the foot on the ground and the tibia fixed.
**Piriformis** acts as an abductor, lateral rotator, and extensor of the thigh, and passes through the greater sciatic foramen.
**Obturator internus** acts as a lateral rotator of the thigh and passes though the trochanteric fossa.
**Coccygeus** supports the pelvic and abdominal viscera, and may possibly flex and abduct the coccyx.
**Levator ani** forms the pelvic floor and the roof of the perineum. Its three parts are the ileococcygeus, pubococcygeus, and the puborectalis, which all work

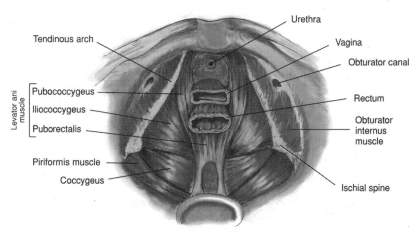

**Figure 1-4**   Pelvic diaphragm

together to slightly flex the coccyx, elevate the anus, and constrict the vagina and the rectum.

**Pelvic diaphragm** (Fig. 1-4) is formed by the levator ani muscles and coccygeus muscle.

**Paracervix:** Region near the cervix. When viewing the cervical os, a **nulli**parous individual will have a *pinpoint* appearance, and a **multi**parous individual will have a *fishmouth* appearance—because of the paracervical tear from delivery or after an artificial dilatation (Fig. 1-5).

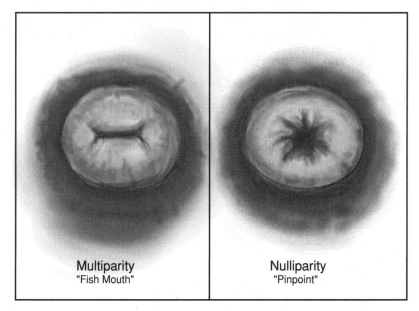

**Figure 1-5**   Cervix

## *EMBRYOLOGY*

| Weeks | *Embryo* Development |
|---|---|
| 1 | Early morula; no organ differentiation. |
| 3 | Double heart recognized. |
| 4 | Initial organogenesis has begun. |
| 6 | *Genetic* sex determined. |
| 8 | Sensory organ development and nondifferentiated gonadal development. |
| | *Fetal* Development |
| 12 | Brain configuration roughly complete, internal sex organs now specific, uterus now no longer bicornuate, and blood forming in marrow. *External* genitalia forming (9 to 12 weeks). |
| 16 | Fetus is active now, sex determination by visual inspection (ultrasound) is possible due to the formed external genitalia. Myelination of nerves, heart muscle well developed, vagina and anus open, and ischium ossified. |
| 20 | Sternum ossifies. |
| 24 | Primitive respiratory movements. |
| 28 | Nails appear and testes at or below internal inguinal ring. |
| 36 | Earlobe soft with little cartilage, testes in inguinal canals, and scrotum small with few rugae. |
| 40 | Earlobes stiffen by thick cartilage, and scrotum well developed. |

# Normal Physiologic Changes in Pregnancy

2

## CARDIOVASCULAR SYSTEM

During pregnancy, the cardiac capacity increases to 70 to 80 ml and cardiac size increases by 12 percent. The stroke volume increases by 25 to 30 percent and reaches its maximum at about 12 to 24 weeks of gestation. The cardiac output increases by 40 percent and reaches its maximum at about 20 to 24 weeks of gestation. There is also an *increase* in the blood volume, RBC mass, oxygen consumption, and plasma volume. There is a *decrease* in blood pressure, peripheral vascular resistance, hematocrit, and hemoglobin. Physical signs may include a late systolic or ejection murmur in 90 to 95 percent of patients due to the increase in stroke volume and 90 percent of women may have normal S3 gallop. There may be reversible changes in the ST, T, or Q waves noted on the ECG due to the left and upward displacement of the heart during pregnancy.

## ENDOCRINE SYSTEM

The average weight gain during pregnancy is 12.5 kg or 27.5 lb. This is due to an increase in breast tissue, increase in blood volume, an increase in water volume, and an increase in uterine contents (about 40 percent of the added weight is from the products of conception). It *is* normal for a pregnant woman to develop *abdominal striae* with pigmentation. The thyroid gland increases in size by 15 percent due to the increased vascularity and glandular hyperplasia. Due to increased levels of estrogen, there is an increase in thyroid binding globulin, T3, and T4 totals but no change in the free circulating T3, T4, and T4 index. Neonatal thyrotoxicosis can be caused by PTU or by thyroid stimulating globulin crossing the placenta, and neonatal hypothyroidism or goiter may be caused by the use of methemazole.

You may consider in hyperthyroidism to check for an increased total T4 level and a decreased TSH. When checking labs, *primary* hyperthyroidism has a decreased TSH, but *secondary* hyperthyroidism has an increased TSH. In hypothyroidism, check for an increase in TSH, and decreased or normal (but decreased free) T3, T4, and T3-resin uptake—treat with thyroid replacement (L-thyroxine).

The pancreas increases its release and production of insulin due to increased levels of estrogen and progesterone. There is also an increase in tissue sensitivity to insulin and an average decrease in the fasting blood sugar levels by 15 mg/dl.

The adrenal gland increases the levels of circulating cortisol to stimulate endogenous glucose production and glycogen storage's and to decrease glucose utilization.

The pituitary increases in size due to chromophobe proliferation in the anterior pituitary, and prolactin production is increased 5- to 10-fold.

## DIGESTIVE SYSTEM

In the gastrointestinal tract, motility decreases due to increased progesterone, and decreased motilin causes a decrease in smooth muscle stimulation. This may account for some of the nausea and vomiting in pregnancy. The increase in acid production in the stomach, the slower emptying time, the increased intragastric pressure, the decreased esophageal peristalsis, and the relaxation of the cardiac sphincter may contribute to the gastroesophageal reflux symptoms noted during pregnancy. The appendix may be displaced to the right flank area, which when inflamed may mimic pyelonephritis. Bilestasis and gallstones may occur due to a slowing in the gallbladder emptying time. The liver is affected by secreting decreased amounts of plasma albumin (about 1 g/dl) and plasma globulins. There is a relative increase in serum alkaline phosphatase because it is secreted by both the liver and the placenta.

## HEMATOLOGIC SYSTEM

Hematologically, there is an increase in the plasma volume up to 50 percent by term, an increase in the blood volume up to 45 to 50 percent by term, and an increase in RBC mass by 30 percent by term even without iron supplementation. In iron deficiency anemia, the pregnant female needs to supplement iron. Therefore, approximately 1000 mg of iron is needed or 325 mg of $FeSO_4$/day. The RBC mass however will increase even more with iron supplementation and the increase is due to an increase in production and not life-span. Therefore, there is an increase in iron need as well. A normal leukocytosis is also noted, primarily due to the increase in the number of polymorphonuclear cells. Also, there is an increase in platelet production and a marked increase in fibrinogen (factor I) and factor VIII, and other clotting factors are also increased, but to a lesser degree (e.g., factors VII, IX, X, and XII).

## RENAL SYSTEM

The kidneys increase in length by 1 to 1.5 cm and the collecting system is more dilated, causing an increase in urinary stasis. The glomerular filtration rate increases by about 50 percent and the renal plasma flow increases by 25 to 50 percent. The renal changes can be attributed to an increase in maternal and placental hormones such as ACTH, ADH, aldosterone, human chorionic somatomammotropin, and thyroid hormone (T3 and T4, but normal free T). The creatinine clearance increases with a peak to about 50 percent by 32 weeks gestation. There is a relative decrease in the serum creatinine and BUN—due to the increased GFR. Also, due to the increased GFR and impaired tubular resorptive capacity, there may be glucose noted in the urine that may not be related to serum levels. Due to the increase in ADH and aldosterone, there is an increase in salt and water retention and increases in renin and angiotensin I and II. The bladder is displaced upward and flattened in anterior-posterior diameter causing an increase in urinary frequency. The bladder capacity is also increased due to an increase in the vascularity and decrease in the muscle tone.

## RESPIRATORY SYSTEM

In the respiratory system, there is enlargement in the nasopharyngeal, tracheal, laryngeal, and bronchial surface areas (due to dilation). Airway resistance is unchanged or decreased in pregnancy. The functional residual capacity, residual volume, and expiratory reserve volume all decrease by 20 percent during pregnancy, while the dead space increases as well as the tidal volume (by 35 to 50 percent) and the inspiratory capacity (by 5 to 10 percent). The increase in the tidal volume and the decrease in the residual volume together cause a marked increase in alveolar ventilation by approximately 65 percent. The minute ventilation increases by 50 percent and the oxygen consumption increases by 15 to 20 percent while the alveolar carbon dioxide decreases due to increased respiratory rate, also known as hyperventilation of pregnancy.

# Normal Obstetric Care

# 3

## DEFINITIONS

**Embryo** refers to the time from conception to about 8 weeks gestation.
**Fetus** is from about 8 weeks to delivery.
**Gravidity** refers to the number of *pregnancies*.
**Parity** refers to the state of giving birth to a fetus, dead or alive, weighing 500 g or more. For example, **G4P3013** means:

| | |
|---|---|
| Gravida | 4 pregnancies |
| Para | 3 full-term births |
| | 0 premature births |
| | 1 abortion |
| | 3 live births (living children) |

**Preterm** refers to being born at any time on or before 37 weeks gestation.
**Immature** refers to an infant weighing between 500 and 1000 g and/or between 20 and 28 weeks gestation.
**Premature** refers to an infant weighing between 1000 and 2500 g and/or between 28 and 37 weeks gestation.
**Mature** refers to an infant weighing greater than 2500 g and/or greater than 37 weeks gestation.
**Postmature** refers to an infant delivered greater than 42 weeks gestation.
**Large for gestational age** (LGA) refers to an infant weighing greater than 4500 g at birth.
**Small for gestational age** (SGA) refers to an infant weighing less than two standard deviations for its gestational age.

11

---
### NUTRITIONAL REQUIREMENTS
---

Pregnant women only need an extra 300 kcal per day for nutrition and post-partum breast feeding women only an extra 500 kcal per day. The normal weight gain during pregnancy should be between 10 and 12 kg or 22 to 27 lb.

---
### INITIAL PRENATAL EVALUATION
---

The initial evaluation should include the following labs:

CBC with differential
Electrolytes
Blood glucose screen
Sickle Cell prep (if indicated)
Rubella titer
VDRL (RPR) titer
Urinalysis with culture and sensitivities
Pap smear and cervical culture
Blood type with complete antibody screening

| Cervical Cultures[a] for | If High Risk Patient |
|---|---|
| GC | Hepatitis B |
| Chlamydia | HIV |
| Group B Streptococcus | TB skin test Toxoplasmosis (if indicated) |

[a]Repeat cultures at 35 to 37 weeks.

---
### COMMON ANTEPARTAL COMPLAINTS
---

The following is a list of complaints commonly encountered during pregnancy:

#### CANDIDA VULVOVAGINITIS
This is caused by *Candida albicans*, and presents as "cottage cheese-appearing" vaginal discharge and irritation, with growth at a pH of 4.5. Treatment includes: anti-fungal agents like fluconazole (1 dose regimen), nystatin, miconazole, and ketoconazole. Also, clotrimazole vaginal suppositories or cream at bedtime for 1 to 2 weeks.

#### PICA
Pica is ingestion of substances with no nutritious value, for example, paint chips or clay. This may be dangerous because of the substitution of nonnutritious bulk for important nutrient food. Pica is associated in patients with chronic, severe iron-deficiency anemia.

### INCREASED URINARY FREQUENCY

Increased urination is due to an increase in vascularity and hormonal changes, and later on it occurs from direct pressure on the bladder.

### SEXUALLY TRANSMITTED DISEASES

#### Syphilis

Syphilis is a STD caused by *Treponema pallidum*, a motile, anaerobic *spirochete*. You may help in the diagnosis by doing a dark-field microscopy of the chancre (by scraping the lesion). A Venereal Disease Research Laboratory (VDRL) test or a Rapid Plasma Reagin (RPR) test is given in a prenatal visit. The causes of a *false-positive test* include: drug use, viral infection, and autoimmune disorders. The specific, confirming test is the fluorescent treponemal antibody absorption test (FTA-ABS). Syphilis can be transmitted to the fetus. This is treated with Benzathine Penicillin G (drug of choice), erythromycin, or ceftriaxone.

#### Chlamydia

Chlamydia is a cause of vulvovaginitis and pelvic inflammatory disease and is associated with an increased incidence of premature labor and premature rupture of membranes (PROM). Chlamydia is treated with a one-day course of Azythromycin or a seven-day course of Erythromycin. Also, Amoxicillin may be substituted in cases of Erythromycin intolerance. Remember to treat any sexual contacts. Infants will receive erythromycin "eye therapy" at delivery.

##### LYMPHOGRANULOMA VENEREUM

This venereal disease is caused by the obligate intracellular parasite, *Chlamydia trachomatis*. It presents as: headache, fever, and a pain**less** vulvovaginal ulcer. The treatment is Tetracycline (if not pregnant) or Erythromycin 500 mg QID for 2 to 3 weeks.

#### Gonorrhea

This is treated with a single dose of IM *Ceftriaxone* (DOC) or Amoxicillin or Spectinomycin (if allergic to penicillin). Since a co-existent chlamydia infection is common, Erythromycin is also added. Do NOT give Tetracycline because of the fetal teeth and bone problems. Tetracyclines can cause teeth to darken. During the second half of pregnancy and during tooth development in a child, AVOID tetracyclines. Also, remember to treat sexual contacts in cases of gonorrhea.

#### Herpes simplex virus

Herpes genitalis is a venereal disease caused by Herpes Simplex Virus type **II**, with the first symptoms occurring 3 to 7 days after exposure. The prodromal symptoms include: *burning*, a visible lesion, *painful* urination, with vesicles and a maculopapular rash. The ulcers (which are *painful*) usually heal in 7 to 10 days. On a *zinc pap smear* there will be *multinucleated giant cells*. (Perform a Hank's smear.) Herpes is treated with topical Acyclovir to improve symptoms. Oral or parenteral treatment is reserved for immunocompromised patients. Vaginal delivery is possible if there are NO active lesions; cesarean section is recommended if active lesions are present. But, viral shedding can still occur even with no visible lesions.

### Human papilloma virus

The HPV 16, 18, 31, 33, and 35 are associated with more malignant problems, like cervical neoplasia. There is a strong association between HPV and *cervical carcinoma*. HPV 6 and 11 are relatively benign, and are associated with *cervical condyloma* and *genital warts* (HPV is the cause of condyloma and koilocytosis with a perinuclear halo). *Condylomata acuminata* are *papillomatous* lesions or venereal warts from the Human *Papilloma* Virus—especially types 16 and 18. HPV 16 and 18 are also associated with noninvasive and invasive *cervical neoplasia*. Treatment includes: 50 percent and 80 percent Trichloracetic acid applied to the lesions bid 3 days/week for 3 weeks, or Podophyllin 25% in benzoin (treat *directly* to the lesion and wash off in 6 to 8 h—since these treatments will destroy infected and *normal* tissue). Podophyllin can cause fetal death or premature labor, so avoid using it during pregnancy. If after 4 to 6 weeks of treatment the lesions persist, then consider cryosurgery, cauterization, or cutaneous laser therapy. None of the "treatments" eradicate the virus. Consider cesarean section for delivery if there are growing lesions present at the vagina.

### Human immunodeficiency virus (HIV)

An HIV infection leads to the development of AIDS. It is transmitted sexually through bodily secretions and can be transmitted from the mother to the infant. The RNA retrovirus has specific surface proteins (gp120 and gp41) and core proteins (p18 and p24) that are detected during serology laboratory diagnosis. The ELISA test is positive and is confirmed with a positive Western Blot test. There is also a positive HIV antigen test and a positive HIV culture. Any pregnant woman who is at risk of having HIV should be screened. NOT all infants who are delivered by HIV-positive mothers contract the virus (particularly if treated with preventive AZT). Only about one-fourth to one-third of the fetuses acquire HIV from vertical transmission from the mother.

### Molluscum contagiosum

This may occur through direct or indirect contact. The infection causes a mild pruritus and multiple painless nodules of *dome-shaped* lesions. These lesions may *spontaneously* resolve. If not, probe the caseous content from the lesion, then apply *carbonic acid*, trichloroacetic acid, or silver nitrate to remove the papules.

### Chancroid

This is a very contagious disease found in *tropical climates*, and is caused by the bacterium *Haemophilus ducreyi*. It presents with a *painful* vulvar ulcer (to the touch) with a foul *odor*. Diagnosis is made by gram stain, culture, and biopsy. The treatment is Erythromycin 500 mg QID for 7 days, or Ceftriaxone.

### Granuloma inguinale

This is caused by the bacterium *Donovania granulomatis*. It is more common in Africa, and presents as a papule that develops into a painless genital ulcer, and on tissue smear examination, "Donovan bodies" (encapsulated bipolar bacteria) can be found. Treatment includes: Tetracycline 500 mg q6 h for 10 to 21 days (caution in early pregnancy due to teeth and bone problems in the developing fetus).

## VAGINITIS

### Trichomoniasis (trichomonas vaginitis)

This is considered another STD found in 20 to 30 percent of pregnant women. The discharge may be *greenish*, frothy, and *foul smelling*. This causes a *strawberry cervicitis*. Flagellated, pear-shaped, motile organisms are seen on the saline wet mount under the microscope. Treatment is with Flagyl (Metronidazole) at a 2 g one time dose but is NOT given in the first trimester—because it can be teratogenic. An alternative is Clindamycin vaginal cream.

### Candidiasis

Candidiasis is caused by the yeast *Candida albicans* and occurs in up to 50 percent of pregnant females. This is NOT a STD (normal flora in women). The discharge may be white and cheesy or curd-like and vaginal itching and burning usually accompanies it. Hyphae and budding yeast are usually seen on the potassium hydroxide wet mount under the microscope. Treatment of choice is one of the antifungal vaginal creams like Monistat, Nystatin or Terazol but may use Diflucan one time oral dosing in isolated cases.

### Gardnerella vaginosis

Gardnerella vaginosis is also quite common. The discharge is usually copious and *gray*, with a *fishy* odor. *Clue cells* (epithelial cells with bacteria) are usually seen with a saline *wet mount* under the microscope. Treatment of choice is with Flagyl or Metrogel (Metronidazole gel) once a day for 5 to 7 days or BID for 7 days. *Gardnerella vaginalis* is an STD that produces this malodorous discharge that itches and burns (in less than 1 of 5 patients).

## BACTERIAL INFECTIONS

### Urinary tract infections (UTIs)

UTIs are the most common medical complications of pregnancy. They are possibly due to hormonal changes and urinary stasis. A urinalysis will show bacteriuria, pyuria, and possibly hematuria. The most common bacterial organism is *Escherichia coli*; other isolated organisms include: *Proteus mirabilis, Klebsiella pneumoniae,* and *Group B streptococcus.* Treat with a week to 10 days of Ampicillin or a Cephalosporin (such as Keflex). Acute pyelonephritis may occur and appear as *flank pain,* fever, vomiting, dehydration, and possibly lead to septic shock. Pyelonephritis requires hospitalization for IV antibiotics.

### Group B streptococcus (GBS)
GBS is considered a part of the normal flora of the GI and can be transmitted to the genital tract by sexual transmission or by *fecal contamination.* The organism is determined by *culture.* The GBS is transferred from the mother to the infant at delivery. This GBS sepsis is the most common *neonatal sepsis.* It is also the second most common cause of bacteriuria. Treat with Ampicillin, Penicillin, or Erythromycin. Due to the infant morbidity and mortality associated with GBS, prenatal cultures are done initially in pregnancy and repeated at 36 weeks. If a positive culture is obtained, then treatment is indicated. See Fig. 3-1.

### Tuberculosis
A positive purified protein derivative (PPD) test means that the patient has had a TB infection in the past (it is NOT necessarily an active disease). You should do a pre-screen on *high*-risk patients in the lower socioeconomic areas or immigrants. There is a risk of congenital tuberculosis with lower birth weight, respiratory distress, and death of the fetus. Therefore, we treat a mother who has the *active disease* during pregnancy with Isoniazid (INH) and vitamin B6. Chest x-ray a patient (shield the abdomen area); if it is positive, take sputum cultures and if these are positive then treat. The idea is that if you do not treat active TB, there is a greater risk to *both* the mother and the fetus.

## PARASITIC INFECTIONS

### Toxoplasmosis
*Toxoplasma gondii* is the cause of the systemic disease toxoplasmosis. Many women (about 1 out of 3) have IgG antibodies against toxoplasmosis and are immune to infection. The parasite is acquired by breathing/exposure to the feces of an infected cat, and by eating contaminated/uncooked meats and dairy products. Therefore, pregnant women should not change the litter box and should avoid coming in contact with cat feces. Fetal infection in the first trimester has the worst prognosis, and the risk for transmission increases through each trimester. The classic triad consists of: (1) hydrocephalus; (2) intracranial calcifications; and (3) chorioretinitis. Diagnosis of congenital infection is: IgM is detected in the cord blood, and placental culture is positive. It is considered a self-limiting disease, but can be treated with pyrimethamine and sulfadiazine (risk of fetal problems). Remember, *prevention* is the best recommendation.

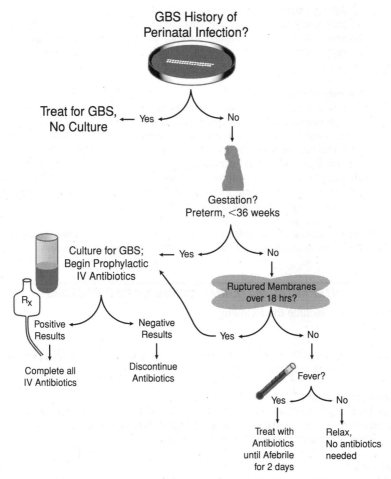

**Figure 3-1**    Management of Group B beta-Hemolytic Streptococcus (GBS)

## VIRAL INFECTIONS

### Rubella

German measles (Rubella) is a ssRNA *togavirus* that can be diagnosed by the appearance of an increase in the HAI *titer* or the appearance of IgM in the *cord blood*. Fetal risk of *Congenital Rubella Syndrome* (CRS) increases if the mother is infected in the *first* trimester (only approximately a 1 percent risk in the second and third trimester). CRS can include: congenital *deafness*, cardiac malformations, retinopathy or other eye lesions, CNS problems, hepatitis, hepatosplenomegaly, and thrombocytopenic purpura. Rubella vaccine is NOT recommended during pregnancy since it is a *live* vaccine (MMR). There is NO treatment recommended. A non-immune mother should be vaccinated after the delivery (postpartum vaccination is NOT contraindicated with breast feeding.)

### Cytomegalovirus (CMV)

This is a herpes DNA virus that is transmitted by sexual contact, through breast milk, and other fluids. CMV is the most common congenital viral infection. An infection presents as a *mononucleosis-like* illness. The risk of maternal-infant transmission is about 40 to 50 percent. The infant may develop: intrauterine growth retardation, *chorioretinitis*, microcephaly, or be asymptomatic, but may lead to mental retardation and other sensory losses. Prevention is important, and proper hygiene and transfusion donor blood testing are recommended.

Other minor complaints include: varicose veins, edema, joint pain, backache, pelvic pressure, round ligament pain, leg cramps, and breast soreness.

## ANTEPARTAL MATERNAL COMPLICATING FACTORS

These factors include the following:

### DRUG ABUSE

Abuse of drugs such as heroin or methadone may cause fetal withdrawal and cocaine or crack may cause placental abruption.

### CIGARETTE SMOKING

Smoking may cause an increased incidence of low birth weight infants or intrauterine growth restriction, increased fetal death or damage in utero, and an increased risk of placental abruption or previa.

### ALCOHOL

Alcohol use may cause an increase in fetal withdrawal symptoms and an increased risk of fetal alcohol syndrome (incidence of 1 in 1500 to 1 in 600 live births) with growth retardation, facial dysmorphology like microcephaly and microphthalmia, and CNS deficits. There may be evidence to support a dose effect relationship due to improved neonatal outcome associated with decreased intake by the third trimester. "Binge" drinking is particularly harmful to the fetus.

## ANTEPARTAL FETAL SURVEILLANCE

### FETAL MOVEMENT COUNTS

The fetal movement counts are based on maternal perception. The assumption is that fetal movements occur if there is adequate fetal oxygenation. This form of surveillance should be initiated when fetal viability is reached. Normally, there should be at least ten movements in twelve hours. If this does not occur or it takes twice as long for ten movements to be counted then the physician should perform a non stress test to monitor the fetus more closely. Over 90 percent of high risk patients will have normal movement counts. Fetal death will occur in 10 to 30 percent of patients who report abnormal counts if no further intervention is done. Due to the advent of more advanced testing, fetal demise is rare and the rate of fetal distress during labor is less than 5 percent.

## NONSTRESS TESTS

These tests are a form of electronic fetal monitoring that monitor the fetal heart rate that has a normal range of 120 beats per minute to 160 beats per minute. The nonstress test, or NST, is based on the fact that fetal body movements are associated with an increase in the fetal heart rate known as accelerations. This suggests that the uteroplacental unit is functioning properly. A reactive NST is defined as a fetal heart tracing strip that has at least two accelerations of the fetal heart rate, each at least fifteen beats above the baseline, lasting for at least fifteen seconds within a twenty minute period. It is felt that a fetus is more active 1 to 2 h after meals and may be less active during sleep cycles, which normally last 20 to 45 min and may increase with fetal age, or with maternal ingestion of drugs or alcohol. Most non-reactive NSTs will become reactive within 45 min; if this does not occur then further testing is required.

## CONTRACTION STRESS TEST OR OXYTOCIN CHALLENGE TEST

This test is an advanced form of monitoring, which monitors the fetal heart rate and its relationship to uterine contractions. To be an adequate test, there must be 3 to 5 contractions in a 10 minute period. Fetal well-being is assessed by the presence or absence of decelerations of the fetal heart rate. If the test is positive, that is presence of fetal heart late decelerations are noted in relation to contractions, there is thought to be some form of fetal compromise, and further evaluation or delivery is required. This test can be categorized as either reactive or non-reactive as with the NST. *Negative* means there are no late decelerations. *Equivocal* means there are non-repetitive late decelerations. *Hyper-stimulation* means that there is greater than five contractions in ten min or contractions lasting more than ninety seconds with evidence of late decelerations following coupled contractions. *Positive* means that there are late decelerations occurring with each of the three contractions in the ten minute time period (refer to Fig. 3-4). If the test is considered negative then it can be repeated once a week as indicated. If the test is considered equivocal or hyperstimulatory then it should be repeated within a 24-h period. A positive test indicates fetal distress or compromise and further evaluation or delivery is indicated. This form of testing is contraindicated in patients predisposed to uterine rupture as with classical C-sections or previous full thickness uterine incisions, or in those predisposed to premature delivery as with premature rupture of membranes, pre-term labor, multiple gestation, incompetent cervix, or polyhydramnios. Also, it is contraindicated in those patients with a predisposition to bleeding as in placenta previa, unexplained vaginal bleeding, or evidence of placental abruption.

## BIOPHYSICAL PROFILE

This is another advanced form of testing that requires the use of the NST and the ultrasound. It is based on the fetal heart rate, breathing movements, limb movements, trunk attitude and movements (tone), and the amniotic fluid volume. The scoring range is from 0 to 2 for each element listed above, with a total score of 10 being the highest. Two points will be given for each positive parameter; therefore a reactive NST gets two points, an amniotic fluid volume of 2 cm or more in all four equal quadrants will receive two points, one to two breathing episodes lasting for at least 30 seconds will get two points, three discreet limb movements equals a score of two, and one extension of the trunk followed by one flexion of the trunk equals two points. If the results of the test are between 0 and 2 then immediate delivery due to possible fetal jeopardy is recommended (75 to 100 percent correlation). A score between 4 and 6 requires that the test be repeated within 24 h or deliver if indicated. A score of 8 to 10 is considered a negative test and fetal well-being has been established; the test can be repeated once a week as indicated. This form of testing has a false positive rate of less than 30 percent.

## FETAL HEART RATE MONITORING

There are two types of fetal heart rate monitoring:

### EXTERNAL MONITORING

This uses ultrasound doppler, which monitors the heart rate through sound waves. Other external techniques include direct fetal echocardiography or phonocardiography but the doppler use is widespread.

### INTERNAL MONITORING

This consists of placing a spiral electrode on the fetal scalp to directly monitor the heart rate; this is also called *direct fetal electrocardiography*.

The baseline fetal heart rate ranges from 120 to 160 beats per minute. The amplitude fluctuations of 5 to 15 beats per minute superimposed on the baseline is known as the fetal heart rate beat to beat variability. This is considered to be a sign of good autonomic system interplay and fetal well being. (Note: the fetal circulation includes the highest $P_{O_2}$ in the *umbilical vein*, and the highest $P_{CO_2}$ in the *umbilical artery*. The *uterine* vein has *mixed* blood, and a *higher* $P_{CO_2}$ than the *umbilical vein*.)

The heart rate transitory changes consist of accelerations and decelerations:

#### Accelerations

These occur as an elevation of the fetal heart rate above the baseline. These are considered to be very reassuring unless associated with decreased variability or development of late decelerations.

#### Decelerations

These occur as a fall of the fetal heart rate below the baseline and are described in relation to contractions. There are three types of decelerations of fetal heart rate: variable decelerations, early decelerations, and late decelerations.

### VARIABLE DECELERATIONS (SEE FIG. 3-2)

These occur as a drop of 10 to 60 beats below the baseline and their behavior pattern is variable in relation to contractions. They don't always have a uniform shape and their amplitude can vary. Decelerations at *variable time* are usually seen in *umbilical cord compression* and are not related to fetal acidosis unless episodes become frequent and prolonged. Remember, cord compression causes a ***variable deceleration***. Compressing the umbilical cord increases the blood pressure of the fetus and decreases the heart rate (with a decreased blood pH and increased $P_{CO_2}$; *respiratory* acidosis). Reposition the mother to relieve the compressed cord.

### EARLY DECELERATIONS (SEE FIG. 3-3)

These occur as a drop of 10 to 40 beats below the baseline, occurring at the same time as the contraction, and are usually seen during normal labor. They usually don't drop below 100 beats per minute and don't

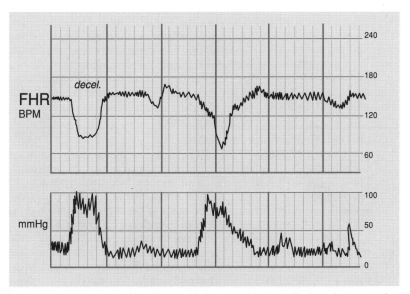

**Figure 3-2  Variable decelerations** may be caused by umbilical cord compression. This causes an increase in the fetal blood pressure and a decrease in the heart rate (bradycardia). Changing the mother's position generally relieves the cord compression and the decelerations.

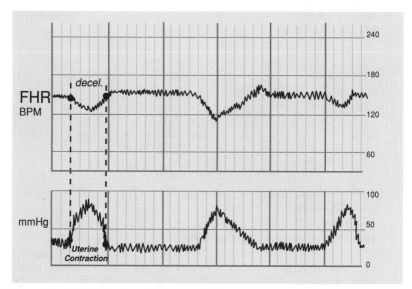

**Figure 3-3   Early Deceleration.** Notice that the deceleration begins and ends at the *same* time as the uterine contraction. The normal fetal heart rate (FHR) is between 120–160 bpm. In the example above, there are three contractions and decelerations.

last longer than 90 seconds. Their shape is uniform and reflects the uterine pressure. These are usually associated with normal *head compression* due to the uterine contractions causing a reflex bradycardia. The *early* decelerations may be due to *head compression* or *fetal hypoxia*. The decelerations usually occur at the *same time* as the contraction— due to *head compression*. This is an ***early deceleration***. (These do NOT cause fetal distress.)

### Late decelerations (SEE FIG. 3-4)
These occur as a drop of 5 to 60 beats below the baseline that occurs after the contraction with a greater lag time than early decelerations. These are usually uniform in shape but the fetal heart rate does not return to baseline until after the end of the contraction, that is the nadir of the deceleration occurs after the apex of the contraction. Late decelerations are thought to be due to factors influencing *uteroplacental gas exchange* such as in fetal *hypoxia (uteroplacental insufficiency)*, *shock* or fetal *metabolic* acidosis. They last less than 90 seconds and are associated with a normal fetal heart rate baseline. They are decelerations that occur *after* the contractions—due to *hypoxia*. This causes a ***late deceleration***. The treatment includes: tocolytics, 100% oxygen, assessment for delivery, and repositioning the mother.

There are several sustained heart rate changes to consider as well:

### SHORT-TERM VARIABILITY
This is the beat to beat variability. As discussed earlier, this is one sign of fetal well-being.

### TACHYCARDIA
A sustained fetal tachycardia where the baseline is *above* **160** beats per minute is usually associated with maternal fever, maternal hyperthyroidism, amnionitis, or fetal hypovolemia. It may also be associated with fetal hypoxia, fetal tachyarrythmia, or parasympatholytic or sympathomimetic drugs. The two ranges are **moderate**, 161 to 180, and **marked**, greater than 180. *Fetal tachycardia may be an early sign of fetal distress.*

### BRADYCARDIA
A sustained fetal bradycardia is when the fetal heart rate baseline is *below* **120** beats per minute, and is usually associated with maternal hypothermia or maternal use of beta adrenergic blocking medications. The two ranges are **moderate**, 100 to 119, and **marked**, less than 100. It is also seen in association with congenital cardiac conduction deficits especially in association with maternal systemic lupus erythematosis. If a *sinusoidal pattern* is demonstrated on the monitoring strip, then *extreme fetal jeopardy* is evident. This is seen in association with fetal anemia and Rh iso-immunization from the fetomaternal transfusion syndrome or with the maternal administration of narcotics.

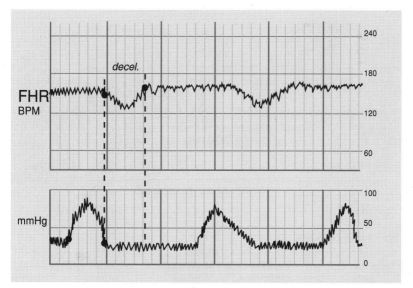

**Figure 3-4   Late Deceleration.** Notice that the deceleration begins at the *end* of the uterine contraction. In the example above, there are three contractions and two decelerations.

## FETAL IMAGING

Ultrasonography is the most widely utilized technique for determination of the gestational age. It is used to estimate fetal weight, to look at fetal growth parameters, fetal anatomy, and amniotic fluid volume, and is in the biophysical profile to access fetal well-being. The most accurate measurements for dating are between 20 and 24 weeks gestation and become less accurate after 30 weeks. To assess fetal gestational age, measurements of the biparietal diameter, femur length, and abdominal circumference are best calculated for ages between 20 and 30 weeks gestation. If the gestational age is between 5 and 12 weeks then a fetal crown rump length is measured.

## GENETIC SCREENING

Genetic screening should be offered to women greater than 35 years old or those with abnormal genetic pedigrees. There are three types of genetic screening tests available: *chorionic villi sampling, amniocentesis,* and a *triple check.* All three tests screen for Down's syndrome and Trisomy 18.

Chorionic villi sampling is usually done between 9 and 11 weeks and has an approximately 2 percent risk of procedural fetal loss.

An amniocentesis can be done between 11 and 14 weeks (early) or between 16 and 18 weeks (standard), and with ultrasound guidance techniques the risk of complications is less than 1 percent. This test can also be used to determine fetal lung maturity when done at a later gestional age and the fluid can be cultured to rule out an amniotic infection.

A maternal multiple markers screen, or triple check, tests the levels of alpha-fetal protein, estriol, and human chorionic gonadotropin in the maternal blood stream. This test is usually done between 16 and 18 weeks gestation on all patients (especially if the α-fetoprotein or AFP is elevated because of its high correlation with open *neural tube defects*).

## INTRAPARTUM

## NORMAL COURSE OF LABOR

The normal course of labor has three stages: first, second, and third.

### FIRST STAGE OF LABOR

The first stage begins at the onset of labor (rupture of membrane, cervical effacement and early dilatation, start of contractions, etc.) and ends with complete dilatation of the cervix with contractions usually coming every 2 to 3 min and lasting 30 to 45 seconds. The variables that influence the first stage of labor include: maternal parity, contraction frequency and duration, dilatation and effacement of the cervix, fetomaternal pelvic diameters, and fetal presentation and position. The first stage of labor has *two phases*: the latent phase and active phase. The *first* stage is usually the *longest* stage of labor and usually lasts an average of 8 to 12 h in primigravids and 6 to 8 h in multigravids.

### Latent phase
The latent phase begins at the onset of regular uterine contractions and ends when the cervix is dilated to three or more centimeters. During the latent phase, the contractions become coordinated, and the cervix softens and effaces.

### Active phase
The active phase begins when the cervix is dilated to three or more centimeters and ends with complete cervical dilatation. During the active phase, the cervix dilates, the presenting part descends, and the cardinal movements of labor begin.

## SECOND STAGE OF LABOR
The second stage of labor begins at the full dilatation of the cervix and ends with the delivery of the infant. This stage can vary from a few minutes to about a couple of hours with an average of 50 min in primiparas and 20 min in multiparas. This stage is dependent upon the fetal presentation and position, fetomaternal pelvic relationships, maternal pelvic soft tissue resistance, the frequency, intensity, duration, and regularity of contractions, and maternal pushing efforts.

## THIRD STAGE OF LABOR
The *final* stage begins at the delivery of the infant and ends with the delivery of the placenta. The length of the stage depends upon the rapidness of placental separation and the means of placental delivery.

---

## ABNORMALITIES OF LABOR

## PROLONGATION OF THE LATENT PHASE
This occurs when there is an increase beyond 20 h in primiparas and beyond 14 h in multiparas. This is usually due to analgesics or hypo/hypertonic uterine contractions. Management is usually supportive therapy with rest and sedation.

## ABNORMAL ACTIVE PHASE
The active phase is considered abnormal either if it is prolonged or if there is an arrest of cervical dilatation for more than 2 h. This is usually associated with an inadequate pelvis, with the gynecoid and anthropoid being the most favorable types (see Fig. 3-7), an abnormal fetal orientation, increased fetal size, or inadequate contractions. Management here must become more invasive either through the use of oxytocin to augment labor or through an operative delivery.

### ABNORMAL *SECOND* STAGE OF LABOR

The second stage of labor becomes abnormal if there is an arrest of descent of the presenting part. It will have similar causes as an abnormal active phase does and management is also invasive, requiring an operative vaginal delivery, with a vacuum or forceps, or a C-section.

### ABNORMAL *THIRD* STAGE OF LABOR

The third stage of labor becomes prolonged if there is an *abnormal placentation* or a delay in separation. There are three such types:

#### Placenta accreta

When the placenta adheres to the myometrium without an intervening decidual layer, with an *accreta vera* being when the villi adhere to the superficial myometrium.

#### Placenta increta

When the depth of invasion of the villi goes deeper into the myometrium.

#### Placenta percreta

When the villi invade the entire myometrial thickness.

The management for third stage abnormalities is manual placental removal, uterine curettage, and in severe instances, hysterectomy. Abnormal placentation is associated with previous history of uterine surgery as in a C-section, placenta previa, grand multiparity, previous uterine curettage, and previously treated Asherman's syndrome (this occurs with vigorous puperal curettage with complete removal of the endometrium, especially when infected, that causes healing by formation of intrauterine adhesions that could possibly lead to amenorrhea and secondary sterility).

---

## CERVICAL EXAMINATION

There are three parts to the cervical exam during labor:

### DILATATION OF THE CERVIX

This is expressed in centimeters and indicates the *diameter*. The range of dilatation is 0 (closed) to 10 cm (complete dilation).

### EFFACEMENT OF THE CERVIX

This refers to how thinned out the cervix is due to its retraction. This is expressed in percentages with 0 percent meaning no effacement and 100 percent meaning completely effaced.

### STATION

Level of the presenting part refers to the station. It consists of seven levels in reference to the pelvic inlet and the ischial spines. These levels are listed below (Fig. 3-5).

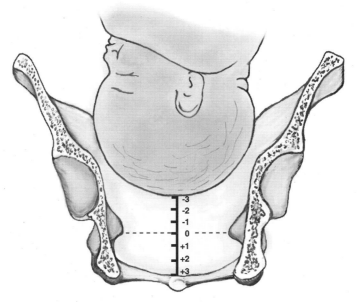

**Figure 3-5**    Fetal Head Stations.

| Level | Placement |
|-------|-----------|
| −3 | presenting part at level of pelvic inlet |
| −2 | ⅓ distance from pelvic inlet to ischial spines |
| −1 | ⅔ distance from pelvic inlet to ischial spines |
| 0 | at level of ischial spines |
| +1 | ⅓ distance below ischial spines |
| +2 | ⅔ distance below ischial spines |
| +3 | presenting part at level of perineum |

## PRESENTATION

There are *three* ways in which the fetus may present during labor: Vertex or cephalic presentation, transverse lie, and breech.

### VERTEX OR CEPHALIC PRESENTATION

This means that the presenting part is the fetal *head.* This type of presentation deals with the relationship of the *occipital* part of the fetal head in the pelvis. This

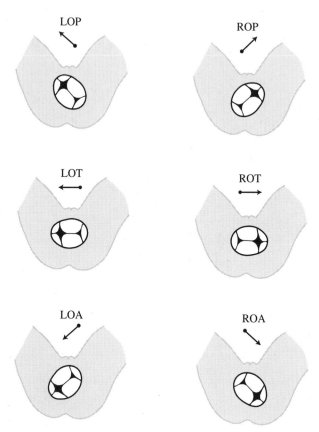

**Figure 3-6**   Vertex Presentations.

is further described as to whether the occiput is in the *right* or *left* position either *anteriorly* or *posteriorly*, whether it is in the right or left position *transversely*, or whether it is in the direct anterior or posterior position (see Fig. 3-6).

### TRANSVERSE LIE
This means that the fetus is lying transversely in the uterus. If attempts at version or rotation fail, then a C-section is indicated in this type of presentation.

### BREECH
Breech presentation occurs when the buttocks or lower extremities present into the mother's pelvis (3 percent of all deliveries). There are *three* types of breech presentation:

#### Frank breech
(65 percent of all breech presentations) In frank breech, the infant's knees are extended and the thighs are flexed, and the infant is almost always delivered via C-section.

### Complete breech

(25 percent of all breech presentations) Complete breech infants have both knees and thighs flexed, and may be delivered vaginally with an experienced obstetrician or by C-section.

### Footling (Incomplete) breech

(10 percent of all breech presentations) The footling breech presentation occurs when there is flexion at the knee and thigh of one side and the other side is extended. These are usually delivered by C-section.

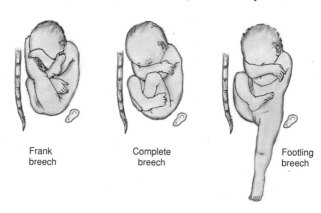

Frank          Complete          Footling
breech         breech            breech

---

## PELVIC INLET (Fig. 3-7)

There are *four* basic pelvic types. It is important to recognize the different *transverse* diameters. Furthermore, the *widest* diameter of the inlet is the posterior area of the *android* or the *anthropoid* pelvis. The pelvic shape is based on the *bony* architecture. The "classic" female type of pelvis is the *gynecoid* ("gyne" = female, and found in 50 percent of women). The *android* pelvis is the "male" type of pelvis (30 percent of women). The shape of the anthropoid pelvis is similar to an ape's and makes up around 20 percent of women's pelvises. Finally, the *platypelloid* is the "flattened" female pelvis (this is fairly rare).

---

## CARDINAL MOVEMENTS OF LABOR

There are *six* cardinal movements of labor in the vertex presentation of normal vaginal deliveries. **Engagement** starts late in pregnancy or at the onset of labor and the most common presentation is the *occiput posterior*. **Flexion of the head** usually aids in engagement and descent. **Descent of the head** usually progresses slowly and depends on the pelvic structure of the mother and the cephalopelvic relationship. **Internal rotation** takes place during descent and usually causes the head to rotate transversely and then anteriorly or posteriorly to get past the ischial spines. **Extension of the head** begins when the head is beneath the symphysis, and is completed with the delivery of the head.

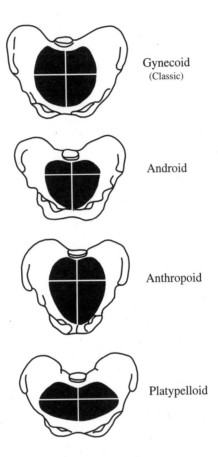

Gynecoid
(Classic)

Android

Anthropoid

Platypelloid

**Figure 3-7**    Pelvic Forms.

**External rotation** occurs after the head has been delivered. The head will rotate to the original position during engagement and then the shoulders will descend in the path similar to that of the head.

## DELIVERY COMPLICATIONS

There are several types of delivery complications. Each type is described below, along with its management.

### COMPOUND PRESENTATION

This is the prolapse of a fetal extremity alongside the presenting part into the lower uterine segment. The most common form is the prolapse of the hand in the cephalic presentation and prolapse of the upper extremity in the breech presentation. Compound presentation occurs **1 in 1200 pregnancies** and can be complicated by umbilical cord prolapse due to the presenting part being unable to be well applied to the cervix during labor. It may be associated with perinatal mortality rates approaching 25 percent. These cases may be delivered vaginally if the infant is term with cephalic presentation and a prolapsed hand or if the infant is premature and gentle replacement can be done without fetal or maternal compromise. A C-section is preferred in cases of premature infants in breech presentation or if presentation is cephalic and compounded by foot or by both a hand and foot.

### SHOULDER DYSTOCIA
This is the inability to deliver the shoulders after the head has been delivered with use of routine obstetrical maneuvers. Usually the chin applies tightly to the perineum as the anterior shoulder becomes impacted behind the symphysis pubis. The total incidence is 0.20 to 0.40 percent of all deliveries, with 0.15 percent if the birth weight is >2500 g and 1.7 percent if the birth weight is >4000 gm. In normal spontaneous vaginal deliveries the rate is around 0.16 percent and it increases to 4.6 percent in attempted mid forceps deliveries. True dystocia may be due to cephalopelvic disproportion. Pseudo-dystocia may be seen with short umbilical cords, abdominal or thoracic enlargement from a tumor, locked or conjoined twins, or with uterine constriction rings. There is an increased risk associated with obese females, maternal gestational diabetes mellitus, small maternal pelvis, post dates, advanced maternal age, and maternal weight gain. There may be complications in up to 50 percent of the cases, causing *birth asphyxia* with related fetal death, neonatal death, or neurologic damage and/or *traumatic injury*. Birth asphyxia may lead to short term sequelae such as metabolic acidosis, shock, renal failure, CNS depression, and seizures and long term sequelae such as mental retardation, cerebral palsy, learning disabilities, seizure disorders, and speech defects. Traumatic injury may lead to fractures of the humerus or clavicle and injuries to the brachial plexus of the anterior shoulder, also known as **Erb's palsy**. One way of managing shoulder dystocia is with the **McRobert's Maneuver,** which consists of sharp maternal thigh flexion against the abdomen with firm suprapubic pressure. (Note: DO NOT DO FUNDAL PRESSURE, FOR IT MAY CAUSE INJURY TO THE MOTHER AND CAUSE THE SHOULDER TO BECOME MORE IMPACTED!) The **Modified Wood's Maneuver** manages the dystocia by applying pressure to the fetal posterior shoulder in an attempt to rotate the shoulder to an oblique lie to give more room for the anterior shoulder. This technique is most successful with mild dystocias.

### UMBILICAL CORD PROLAPSE
This is the descent of the umbilical cord into the lower uterine segment (ahead of the presenting part). There are *three* types of prolapse:

#### Fundic presentation
The prolapse is below the level of the presenting part before the rupture of membranes and the cord is easily palpated through the membranes if the cervix is dilated.

### Occult cord prolapse

The cord is adjacent to the presenting part, variable decelerations or prolonged bradycardias may be noted on the fetal heart tracing and usually cannot be palpated during pelvic exam.

### Overt cord prolapse

The prolapsed cord is below the presenting part with displacement of the cord into the vagina or introitus common, and usually is associated with rupture of membranes.

Prolapse of the cord is caused by the failure of the presenting part to adequately occlude the lower uterine segment. It is only seen in about 0.18 percent of deliveries. Associated risk factors include: multiparity, prematurity, multiple gestation, malpresentation, artificial rupture of membranes, forceps, fetal scalp electrode placement, and pH sampling. Management is most effective by immediate delivery means.

## OBSTETRICAL OPERATIVE PROCEDURES

### VACUUM-ASSISTED VAGINAL DELIVERY

This is used only in vertex presentation and may be used in instances where the cervix has an anterior lip and is not fully dilated, although complete dilation is recommended. There are two types of vacuum extractors used, the malmstrom extractor and the soft cup extractor. The **malmstrom extractor** has a metal cup attached to a traction handle by a chain with rubber tubing attached to a device for vacuum. This type has several different size ranges and may be used in instances of fetal head malrotation. The **soft cup**, known as the silastic or mityvac, is made of a soft material and only comes in one size. Vacuum extraction is contraindicated when there is a non-vertex presentation, a premature infant, excess fetal scalp sampling, suspected cephalopelvic disproportion, and the fetal position is higher than 0 station. Maternal lacerations, fetal intracranial bleeding, fetal scalp abrasions or lacerations, and fetal cephalohematomas are some of the complications incurred from vacuum use.

### FORCEPS-ASSISTED VAGINAL DELIVERY

This is used only when the cervix is fully dilated. It may be indicated when maternal expulsive efforts are inadequate, in situations of fetal distress, and in fetal rotation and descent disorders. Other conditions that must be present for its use include: membranes should be ruptured; head engaged below +2 station; head in vertex presentation or face presentation with chin anterior (not in brow presentation); or face presentation with chin posterior and in breech presentation if the head is engaged in the occiput anterior position. Also it is important for no suspicion of cephalo-pelvic disproportion (CPD) and the bladder should be empty. There are six classifications of forceps deliveries, which are listed below.

A. *Outlet forceps* require that the fetal scalp be visible without separating the labia, the fetal head is positioned on the perineum, the fetal skull reaches the pelvic floor, and the sagittal suture is in the anteroposterior diameter or in the right or left occiput anterior or posterior position but no more that 45 degrees from the midline.
B. *Low forceps* require that the fetal head be at +2 or more station and the rotation can be less than, equal to, or greater than 45 degrees. The fetal head does not reach the pelvic floor.
C. *Mid forceps* require that the fetal head is engaged but the leading edge is higher than +2 station. This type of delivery is only done in circumstance of fetal or maternal compromise and a C-section should be planned in the event that it fails.
D. *High forceps* is the application of the forceps at any time before the head is engaged. Due to significant risks to the mother and the infant, this maneuver is virtually obsolete in modern obstetrical practice and has been replaced with the C-section mode of delivery.
E. *Failed forceps* is an unsuccessful attempt at forceps delivery and abandonment for a C-section delivery.
F. *Trial forceps* is when tentative and cautious traction is applied with forceps with the intent of abandonment for a C-section delivery if undue resistance is encountered.

We will discuss *four* types of forceps used. The *Tucker-McLane* forceps are used in outlet forceps deliveries where little traction is needed and when there is only minimal fetal head molding or in rotating from occiput posterior to occiput anterior. *Simpson* forceps (or *DeLee-Simpson* or *Elliot*) are used for traction in the occiput anterior position or in one of the oblique anterior positions or in a fetal head with marked molding. *Kielland* forceps are used for rotation purposes such as from occiput posterior to occiput anterior or for transverse arrest. The *Piper* forceps are used for the after-coming head in breech deliveries. Forceps are contraindicated if there is CPD or in situations of significant fetal head molding or caput formation. Most complications from forceps are seen in cases of difficult mid forceps deliveries or high forceps deliveries.

## CESAREAN SECTION DELIVERY (Fig. 3-8)
A *C-section* involves delivery of the fetus through an incision in the *uterus* after abdominal wall incision. ("C-section" refers to the *uterine incision*, NOT the *skin* incision.) This form of delivery is indicated when there is fetal distress, abnormal fetal position as in breech or transverse lie, fetal hydrocephalus or large fetal tumors or anomalies, cephalopelvic disproportion with expected shoulder dystocia, mal-placentations such as previa or abruption, previous maternal history of C-section (sometimes indicated), and at times, may be indicated in maternal illness such as pregnancy-induced hypertension or gestational diabetes mellitus. There are very few contraindications except for those instances of extreme maternal illness making surgery unsafe or in cases of fetal death. The most common complications are those related to post-operative infection (but this has decreased due to the use of pre-operative

antibiotics) and anesthesia complications. Post-operative hemorrhage has decreased due to the use of intra-operative pitocin, methergine, and PGF-2α. Other complications include intra-operative injury to the urinary bladder, reproductive organs, or the bowel.

There are *three classifications* of incisions for C-section (*see Fig. 3-8*):

### Transverse incision
This refers to a transverse cut into the *lower* uterine segment ("Low transverse C-section"). This type of procedure is also known as the *Kerr technique* and is the *most common* type used today due to the *decreased* risk of hemorrhage and uterine rupture in subsequent pregnancies.

### Vertical incision
This is also known as the *Kronig technique*, and refers to a *vertical* incision into the *lower* uterine segment and is the second most common type used ("Low vertical C-section"). This form is recommended in cases of fetal mal-presentation due to the ability to extend the incision if needed, although there is a higher risk of the incision extending to the cervix and of uterine rupture in subsequent pregnancies.

### Classical incision
This term refers to a vertical incision taken superiorly through the upper uterine segment ("Classical C-section"). This procedure is *less* commonly used, but it may be indicated when there is an anterior placenta or placenta previa, a fetal mal-presentation such as transverse lie, a poorly developed lower uterine segment, or if the bladder is unable to be dissected from the cervix. It carries an increased risk of hemorrhage, infection, and subsequent pregnancy uterine rupture.

### CERCLAGE
This is a procedure in which a suture is placed into the cervix to prevent premature dilation in patients diagnosed with an incompetent cervix. Diagnosis can be accomplished by discovering a repeated history of mid-trimester pregnancy losses characterized by premature and painless cervical dilation and effacement, if a number 6 or 8 *Hagar* dilator passes easily into the cervical os in the non-pregnant state, or if there is funneling of the cervical internal os seen by ultrasound, hysteroscopy, or hysterosalpingography. This procedure is contraindicated in cases of already advanced cervical dilation, rupture of membranes, heavy vaginal bleeding, or multiple gestations. Complications include bleeding, infection, rupture of membranes especially if the cervix has already dilated, and pre-term labor due to the cervical manipulation. There are three types of the procedure classified. The *Shirodkar* is a planned procedure often done prior to the onset of pregnancy or in early pregnancy when there is thought to be less bleeding. It involves bladder and posterior fornix dissection with placement of a mersilene suture at the internal cervical os. A *McDonald* cerclage uses mersilene or another non-absorbable suture, and is placed in a *purse-string* fashion around the cervix usually between **14 and 16**

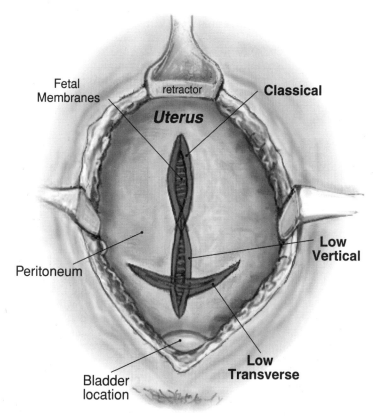

**Figure 3-8**   Types of Cesarean Section.

weeks. This form does not require any form of dissection. Suturing across the cervix to prevent further dilatation (when significant dilatation has already occurred) is known as the *Worm* cerclage, and is not used as often.

### VERSION
This is a process used in fetal mal-presentations. There are *two* types of version classifications:

#### External cephalic version
This version classification is used in the management of singleton breech presentations. If the fetal head is not engaged and the gestation is between 36 and 38 weeks it is more successful; however it can be performed up to 42 weeks of gestation but has a higher failure rate. It is not recommended in the earlier weeks of gestation because there is a higher chance of the fetus returning to the original breech position. It is also

more successful with multiparous females (due to lax abdominal walls), adequate amniotic fluid volume, and either unengaged complete or footling breech presentations. This is used more widely now since the advent of tocolytic therapy. *Contraindications* of external version include (1) if the fetal head is engaged in the pelvis, (2) if there is marked oligohydramnios (or a marked *deficiency* in the volume of amniotic fluid) present, (3) if placenta previa is present, (4) premature rupture of membranes, (5) previous uterine surgery, (6) a suspected or documented congenital malformation, (7) an apparent or suspected intra-uterine growth restriction, (8) frank breech presentation, and (9) due to the use of tocolytics, maternal cardiac disease, diabetes mellitus, and thyroid disease. *Complications from this procedure include:* intra-uterine fetal demise secondary to cord entanglement if done too early in the pregnancy, abruptio placentae, premature rupture of membranes, pre-term labor, umbilical cord prolapse, trans-placental fetomaternal hemorrhage, and uterine rupture.

### Internal podalic version
This is the second type of version classification. The operator places a hand into the completely dilated cervix and grasps both feet of the infant, performs an amniotomy, and applies distal traction to both lower extremities until the feet are delivered out through the vagina, and then proceeds in the routine fashion of a normal breech delivery. *This is rarely performed except in lifesaving situations*, such as fetal distress as in second twin, prolapsed cord, or significant maternal hemorrhage as with early placental separation. The cervix must be completely dilated and membranes intact for this procedure to be done successfully. Due to the severity of the procedure, an intravenous line should be started, the maternal blood should be typed and cross matched, and appropriate anesthesia present. Therefore, this procedure is contra-indicated in rupture of membranes, oligohydramnios, and a partially dilated cervix. Complications include uterine rupture, maternal hemorrhage, fetal intracerebral hemorrhage, birth asphyxia, long bone fetal fracture, fetal joint dislocation, fetal epiphyseal plate separation, and CNS defects.

# POSTPARTUM (OR THE PUERPERIUM)

## PHYSIOLOGIC CHANGES

- The cardiovascular system is affected by an auto-transfusion of 500 ml to 750 ml of blood immediately following delivery and mobilization of the extracellular fluid.
- There is decreased ureteral dilation in the renal system, but in up to 11 percent of postpartum mothers there may be persistent dilation

and persistent post-void residual due to a cystocele. The kidneys should return to their normal functioning state in six weeks, but the time frame may be variable.

• The reproductive system shows changes in the uterus, which begins to involute and decrease in size and volume in the initial six weeks postpartum. The remaining decidua is sloughed off in the initial 7 to 10 days and by day 16 to 18, there should be normal endometrium present. The cervix should retract down to about 1 cm or less. Menses should return at a range of 20 to 120 days in non-breast feeding mothers and ovulation should occur around 45 days postpartum. There may be delays in return of menses and ovulation in mothers who are breast feeding. The breasts are affected by both the anterior and posterior pituitary. If the mother does decide to breast feed, then when the infant suckles, *oxytocin* is released from the *posterior pituitary*, which stimulates myoepithelial cells to contract, causing milk to be released from breast alveoli. **Prolactin** is released from the *anterior pituitary* when the infant is suckling to stimulate *milk **prod**uction* in the breast alveoli. Some women may experience *breast engorgement* within 3 days after delivery, while others may experience nipple soreness or mastitis. The vaginal discharge during the postpartum period is characterized by *three names or phases*:

### LOCHIA RUBRA
This is the blood-tinged discharge containing shreds of tissue and dedidua (*"rubra = red"*).

### LOCHIA SEROSA
This is a paler, more *serous* discharge.

### LOCHIA ALBA
Usually during the second or third postpartum week the lochia becomes thicker, mucoid, and yellowish-white, and consists mostly of leukocytes and degenerated decidual cells (*"alba = white"*).

The bleeding and lochia usually are completed by the fifth week postpartum.

---

## COMPLICATIONS

### POSTPARTUM HEMORRHAGE
The hemorrhage is caused by uterine atony, uterine inversion, coagulation defects, and abnormal placenta problems. Consider the loss of over 500 ml as significant loss that may be from the *spiral arteries* and *decidual veins*, or through *trauma*. Postpartum hemorrhage is classified into two categories:

### Early postpartum hemorrhage
This occurs within 24 h after delivery and is usually caused by placental problems, uterine atony, cervical or vaginal lacerations, uterine rupture, or blood dyscrasias.

### Late postpartum hemorrhage
This occurs anywhere from 24 h to 4 weeks postpartum and is usually caused by retained products of conception.

> NOTE: *Prostaglandins* Oxytocin or $PGF_{2-\alpha}$ may be given to increase the uterine tone in *uterine atony* (increased uterine *contractions*). Remember, $PGF_{2-\alpha}$ is the most potent prostaglandin for contractions (to induce labor), and it stimulates tubal *motility*. $PGE_2$ also causes contraction of the uterus. It *relaxes* the tubal isthmus and allows for the "cervical ripening." $PGE_2$ keeps the ductus arteriosus open.

Types of management include: direct uterine fundal message, use of methergine, pitocin, or $PGF_{2-\alpha}$, transfusion, repair of lacerations, removal of retained products, bilateral iliac artery ligation, and in rare cases hysterectomy.

### LACERATIONS
Lacerations to the cervix, vagina, and perineum can be caused during delivery. There are *four* types of vaginal and perineal lacerations. These are categorized as:

#### First degree
This involves the vaginal mucosa only or perineal skin.

#### Second degree
This involves the underlying fascia or muscle (into the submucosal tissues), but not the rectal sphincter.

#### Third degree
This extends through the anal sphincter, but not into the rectum.

#### Fourth degree
This extends into the rectal mucosa.

### POSTPARTUM INFECTIONS
These may include infections of the genital tract, urinary tract, or breasts. Febrile morbidity is considered to be a temperature greater than 38°C after the first 24 h postpartum. Postpartum endometritis is characterized by tachycardia, a temperature greater than 38.8°C, uterine tenderness, malaise, and profuse and foul-smelling lochia. Pathogens are usually either group A or B beta-hemolytic strep or anaerobes such as bacteroides. To treat, use either a single broad spectrum antibiotic such as cefoxitin, cefotaxime, cefoperozone, moxalactam, or piperacillin, or combination drugs for anaerobes such as an aminoglycoside

and clindamycin, penicillin and chloramphenicol, or an aminoglycoside and metronidazole. Signs and symptoms of acute cystitis may occur on the first or second postpartum day. Most common organisms are the coliform bacteria (such as *E. coli*). A patient with a positive urine culture during pregnancy has a higher risk. Pyelonephritis usually manifests itself on the third or fourth day by the patient exhibiting fever, chills, flank pain, and, frequently, nausea and vomiting. Treatment is with the appropriate antibiotic for the organism isolated, fluid hydration, and good urine drainage. As mentioned earlier, the breast may become engorged, causing a postpartum mastitis to develop. The common bacteria causing postpartum mastitis is *Staphylococcus aureus*, and it can occur from a bite or sucking from the child. It usually lasts for more than one week and the breast is inflamed and painful, and the individual may develop a fever. A *Streptococcus* infection will NOT be pyogenic, but will cause a *cellulitis*. Treatment of mastitis (usually due to penicillin-resistant staphylococcus) is Penicillinase-resistant antibiotics, Methicillin, or Cephalosporins.

## POSTPARTUM CARDIOMYOPATHY
This is a disorder of the heart muscle presenting with the onset of cardiac failure within the first month postpartum but may occur up to 3 to 5 months postpartum. The cause is unknown but it is most commonly seen in older multiparous females without evidence of prior heart disease, females who had pregnancy-induced hypertension or multiple gestations, or it may follow a stillbirth or early abortion. Pathologic findings include focal degeneration and fibrosis of muscle fibers with mural thrombi but no evidence of coronary artery disease. These patients are managed with digitalis and conventional medical management of pulmonary edema, anticoagulation, and bed rest and their prognosis is usually good if the heart size returns to normal within six months. Repeat pregnancy only is recommended in those with normal left ventricular function.

## POSTPARTUM HEMOLYTIC UREMIA
Postpartum *hemolytic uremia* is renal failure due to intra-renal or intra-vascular coagulation. The cause is unknown and it is usually manifested 1 to 10 weeks postpartum. Diagnostic tests include coagulation factors and fibrinogen. Drug therapy for hyperkalemia, hyperuricemia, and hypertension along with digitalis and a transfusion are the usual methods of management.

## POSTPARTUM PREECLAMPSIA
Postpartum *preeclampsia* occurs rarely after 48 h, but can occur up to 14 days postpartum. Pregnancy-induced hypertension (PIH) occurs in 25 percent of antepartum cases, 50 percent of intrapartum cases, and 25 percent of postpartum cases. Late postpartum PIH, which occurs after greater than 48 h, is postulated to be due to retained placental fragments and the patient may need uterine curettage. Preeclampsia is characterized by: *hypertension*, *proteinuria*, edema, coagulopathies, and hyperreflexia. *Eclampsia* includes the development of *seizures*. Treat with vasodilators (for blood pressure control), bed rest, sedation, and magnesium sulfate (for the neurologic problems).

## THROMBOPHLEBITIS

This is thought to be associated with an increase in bed rest postpartum and a decrease in ambulation. There is an increased risk of recurrence with future pregnancies. Thrombophlebitis may lead to a pulmonary embolism and the incidence of superficial thrombophlebitis, deep vein thrombosis, and pulmonary embolism is 2 to 6 times higher in the postpartum period than in the antepartum period. *Deep vein thrombosis* requires IV *heparin* with a doppler ultrasound until the symptoms disappear. Check the PTT, and for Homan's sign—pain when you dorsiflex the foot. Remember, heparin does NOT cross the placental barrier, but *warfarin* does ("war" is bad or teratogenic)—therefore, do NOT give warfarin to a pregnant woman.

## POSTPARTUM DEPRESSION

This depression is thought to be correlated with marked hormonal alterations after delivery and the substantial new burdens and responsibilities that result. This is usually a common disorder that is self-limiting and benign but may be more profound in women with a history of depression before pregnancy and those without an effective support mechanism. Some women may develop a frank psychotic state and require psychiatric treatment.

## POSTPARTUM PNEUMONIA

Postpartum *pneumonia* may manifest itself in females with a history of obstructive lung disease, smoking, and endotracheal intubation. Symptoms include: productive cough, fever, chills, rales, chest pain, and infiltrates. The most common organism is *Mycoplama pneumoniae* or *Streptococcus pneumoniae* and the management is with the appropriate antibiotic, oxygen, and IV fluid hydration.

# Complications of Pregnancy

4

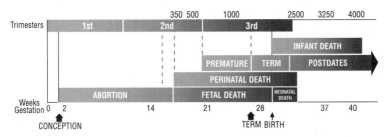

Perinatal Timeline

---

## FETAL LOSS

Fetal losses can happen in any of the three trimesters.

---

## SPONTANEOUS ABORTIONS

These occur in the first two trimesters (up to about 20 weeks gestation), and can be divided into seven types (see Table 4-1).

### MISSED SPONTANEOUS ABORTION
The embryo or fetus dies in utero (before 20 weeks), with *retained* products of conception.

### THREATENED ABORTION
This is defined as when there is intrauterine bleeding (before 20 weeks), *without* expulsion of the products of conception—with or without contractions.

### INEVITABLE ABORTION
This is when there is intrauterine bleeding (before 20 weeks) with *cervical dilation, without* expulsion of the products of conception.

### COMPLETE SPONTANEOUS ABORTION
This occurs when there is intrauterine bleeding (before 20 weeks) with *total* expulsion of the products of conception.

41

#### INCOMPLETE ABORTION

This occurs when there is intrauterine bleeding with expulsion of *some*, but not all, of the products of conception.

#### INFECTED ABORTION

This is defined as when there is an associated *infection* in the genital tract.

#### SEPTIC ABORTION

This is when there is *systemic* dissemination of an *infected* abortion.

## FIRST AND SECOND TRIMESTER LOSSES

First trimester losses occur up to 12 weeks gestation and are called *early spontaneous abortions*. They are usually due to embryological or fetal cytogenetic abnormalities. Almost 50 percent are autosomal trisomies of all chromosomes except chromosome 1 and the most common being trisomy 16, while 20 percent are polyploidy with ¾ being triploidy and ¼ being tetraploidy. The rest of the losses are due to aneuploidy with the single most common being monosomy X, or Turner's syndrome, with 2 percent surviving to term. If the losses are not due to cytogenetic abnormalities they may be due to gross structural anomalies, mendelian genetic problems, or multifactorial genetic problems. If the loss occurs after 12 weeks but before 20 weeks, it is considered a late spontaneous abortion. These second trimester losses are usually due to uterine *anatomic defects* such as uterine septum, submucosal fibroids, and cervical incompetence. *Maternal systemic diseases* such as SLE, diabetes mellitus, and hypothyroidism; *infections* such as syphilis and parvovirus B19; fetal erythroblastosis, fetomaternal hemorrhage, and nonimmune hydrops are also causes of second trimester losses.

The criteria for each type of spontaneous abortion are listed in Table 4-1.

About 75 percent of spontaneous abortions occur before 16 weeks and 62 percent before 12 weeks. Sixty percent of the abortions in the first trimester

**Table 4-1** Characteristics of Varying Types of Abortions

| Criteria | Complete | Incomplete | Inevitable | Threatened | Missed | Septic |
|---|---|---|---|---|---|---|
| Bleeding | variable | yes | yes | yes | **no** | variable |
| Cramping | variable | yes | yes | variable | **no** | variable |
| Cervical dilation | yes | yes | yes | no | **no** | yes |
| Tissue passed | yes | yes | variable | no | **no** | yes |
| Fever | **no** | **no** | **no** | no | **no** | **yes** |

Types of Abortions

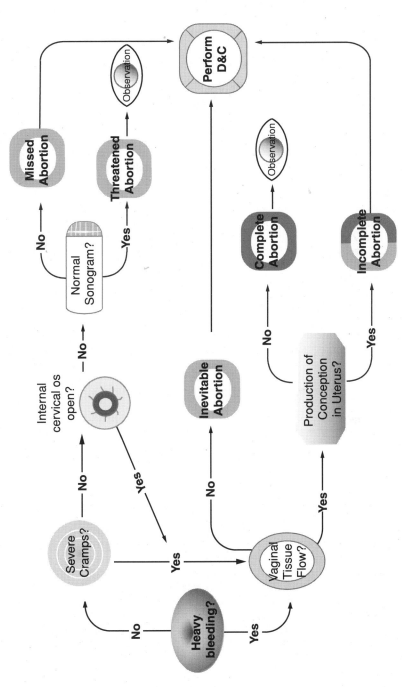

**Figure 4-1**  Management of first trimester bleeding.

43

have abnormal karyotypes with half being aneuploid and half duploid. Of the fertilized ova, 15 percent do not divide, 15 percent are lost before implantation in the first week, 25 percent are lost during implantation in the second week, and 10 percent are lost following the first missed menses. *Genetic abnormalities* top the list of causes responsible and the second leading cause of spontaneous abortions is *unknown*. Other causes include: infection, anatomic defects, endocrine factors, immunologic factors, and maternal systemic disease. Associated risk factors include: couple age, no previous normal pregnancy at term, previous spontaneous abortion history, previous stillbirth history, previous history of infant malformations, previous history of infant genetic defects, medical maternal complications such as diabetes and hyper- or hypothyroid, and parental translocation carriers. An evaluation of a spontaneous abortion may include blood work such as a quantitative β-hCG, a CBC, and a blood type and screen. An ultrasound may be done to look for a gestional sac, fetal pole, and fetal heart motion. It would be also important to rule out other possible causes of bleeding and cramping such as an ectopic, prolonged hyperestrogenism, hydatidiform mole, pedunculated myoma, cervical neoplasia, ruptured tubo-ovarian abscess, and membranous dysmenorrhea. Complications may include hemorrhage, sepsis, disseminated intravascular coagulation, salpingitis, peritonitis, septic shock, thrombophlebitis, embolism, and complications of surgery such as perforation, bowel and bladder injury, and fistula formation. Most types of spontaneous abortions (missed, inevitable, incomplete) will require a D & C; threatened and complete abortions, however, may be managed expectantly and through observation. See Fig. 4-1.

---

## FETAL DEATH

If a pregnancy loss occurs between about 16 and 24 weeks gestation, then it is considered an **intrauterine fetal demise**, **IUFD**, or *fetal death in utero*. This can be discovered early in pregnancy by absence of uterine growth, decreasing β-hCG, and/or 2 negative UCG after having an initial positive test. Later in pregnancy, fetal death is discovered if the mother does not note fetal movement, is not able to document fetal heart tones, or if on ultrasound there is no fetal heart motion, positive clot formation in the fetal heart chambers, or no fetal movement. Also, on other imaging studies due to post-mortem changes in the degenerating fetus, one may see the *Spalding's sign* where there is overlapping skull bones, or *Robert's sign*, where there is gas noted in the great vessels, and/or exaggeration of fetal spinal curvature or spinal angulation. And after 4 to 5 weeks post-mortem there may be a decrease in the fibrinogen. The most common cause of IUFD is idiopathic, seen in about 50 percent of the cases. Other causes include maternal hemorrhage, RBC isoimmunization, cardiac anomalies, chromosomal abnormalities, multiple structural anomalies, viral infections such as HPV B19 and Fifth disease, hematologic diseases such as alpha thalassemia, major fetal anomalies from cardiovascular or CNS, karyotypic/cytogenetic such as monosomy X or trisomies, and TORCH intrauterine infections, listerosis, and parvovirus B19. The two major complications are DIC and depression due to the grief of the loss. See Fig. 4-2 for the

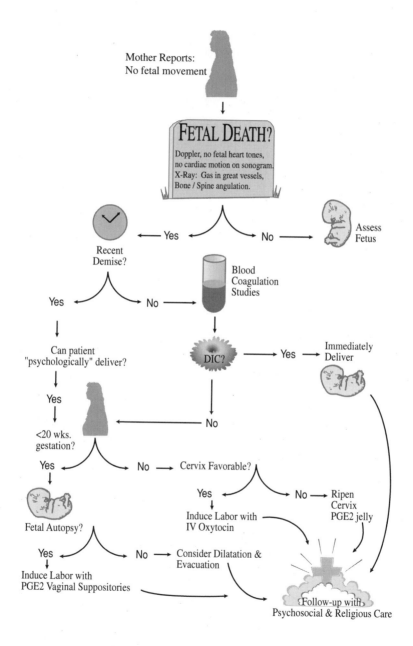

**Figure 4-2**  Management of Fetal Demise

management of these patients. If the cervix is considered to be unfavorable, then it may be ripened with laminaria or dilateria, PGE 2 vaginal suppository or gel, or PGE 1 (cytotec). In a favorable cervix, the labor can just be induced with intravenous pitocin and/or artificial rupture of membranes. If the pregnancy is less than 20 weeks, a D & C can be performed.

## THIRD TRIMESTER LOSSES

A pregnancy loss *after* 24 weeks is considered to be a stillbirth. These losses are usually due to maternal systemic diseases such as hypertension and preeclampsia, maternal environmental factors such as drug abuse or trauma, third trimester bleeding, and IUFDs.

There are several types of third trimester bleeding:

### PLACENTAL ABRUPTION

Placental abruption is defined as *premature separation* of a normally implanted placenta prior to the third stage of labor that is not in the lower uterine segment (Fig. 4-3). The hemorrhage occurs into the desidua basalis and is characterized by *painful bleeding*. This occurs in about 1 of 120 deliveries at term, with fetal death occurring in 1 of 420 deliveries, and 5 to 15 percent will recur. Placental abruption is the most common cause of DIC in pregnancy. Sometimes a *couvelaire uterus*, which is extensive extravasation of blood into the myometrium, may result. PIH or *pregnancy-induced hypertension* is the major cause of placental abruption. Other causes of placental abruption include: trauma, polyhydramnios, cocaine use, smoking, prolonged premature rupture of membranes (PPROM), and a short umbilical cord.

There are *three* types of abruption possible:

### External or overt abruption
This is when the blood is either *bright* red or *dark* red ("port-wine" color) and clotted, and mild pain is experienced unless in labor.

### Internal or concealed abruption
This is defined as when there is *little to no* vaginal bleeding (because the blood is trapped), severe pain, and a hard and very tender uterus. There may be an increased risk of shock.

### Mixed or combined abruption
There is a combination of the concealed and overt types.

The diagnosis is based more on the *clinical aspect* than the laboratory values. Clinical manifestations include contractions, abdominal pain, uterine tenderness, and vaginal bleeding. Some important lab work would include PT, PTT, Fibrinogen, CBC, and Blood Type and Screen. Usually the first values to be affected are the platelets and fibrinogen, which will both drop below normal values. An ultrasound may be useful also since a retroplacental clot may be visualized, but this has a high false negative rate for diagnosis, with only about 20 percent being diagnosed.

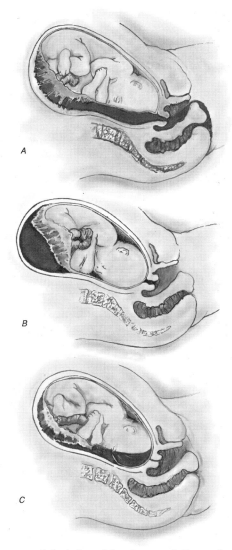

**Figure 4-3**    Three types of abruption of the placenta: *A.* External or overt; *B.* internal or concealed; and *C.* mixed or combined.

Probably the most common risk factors for developing an abruption is whether there has been some form of *maternal trauma* or *maternal drug abuse*, especially cocaine. Other risk factors include short umbilical cord, uterine anomalies, maternal hypertension, smoking, folic acid deficiency, polyhydramnios, inferior vena cava compression, antiphospholipid antibody syndrome, and maternal age.

Complications associated with abruption are: fetal-maternal bleeding, Rh isoimmunization, DIC, fetal hypoxia, shock, acute cor pulmonale, renal cortical and tubular necrosis, transfusion hepatitis, and uterine apoplexy or decreased uterine contractility. These patients should be hospitalized immediately and given oxygen therapy, intravenous fluids, and continuous fetal surveilance, and in the face of a severe abruption, immediate delivery should be the norm.

### PLACENTA PREVIA

*Placenta previa* describes an abnormal placental implantation in the lower uterine segment within the zone of cervical effacement and dilation in advance of the fetal presenting part. This is characterized by *painless bleeding* in the third trimester and there may be an associated history of spotting during the first and second trimesters. There are *four* types of abnormal placental implantation to consider (Fig. 4-4):

#### Total or complete previa
This describes a placenta that completely covers the cervical internal os.

#### Partial previa
The placenta only covers a *part of* the internal os (NOT the entire internal os).

#### Marginal previa
The placenta just reaches, but does not cover any of the internal os of the cervix.

#### Low-lying placenta
This is one that is implanted in the lower uterine segment, but does not cover any of the cervical internal os.

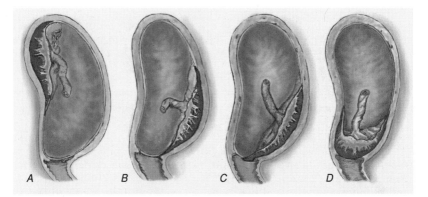

**Figure 4-4**   Placenta Previa. Types of placental implantation: *A*. Normal implantation; *B*. marginal previa vs. low-lying placenta; *C*. partial previa; and *D*. complete previa.

Previas may occur in 1 in 4 pregnancies at 16 weeks with up to 5 percent involved in spontaneous abortions, and in 1 in 200 pregnancies at 40 weeks with 20 percent being total previas and 90 percent found in parous females. It may occur in 1 in 20 pregnancies if the female is grand multiparous. Placenta previas are usually due to scarred or poorly vascularized endometrium in the corpus. A larger placenta or one in a multiple pregnancy has *twice the risk* of becoming a previa and abnormal placental forms such as suscenturiate lobe or placenta diffusa also have an increased risk for previa formation. Other risk factors include advanced maternal age, multiparity, history of previous C-section (*3 times the risk*), and previous history of a placenta previa. Complications include bleeding or hemorrhage which may be due to mechanical separation of the placenta from the implantation site either during cervical effacement and dilation or during lower uterine segment formation or from cervical/intravaginal manipulation. Bleeding may also be due to rupture of venous lakes that are poorly supported in the decidua basalis or from placentitis. Other complications include shock, maternal death, prematurity, perinatal death in 60 percent, fetal hypoxia, birth injury, and fetal hemorrhage. Initially, hospitalization may be required. Some patients are placed on tocolytics unless contracting and bleeding, and on bedrest. Blood replacement may be given to maintain a hematocrit of 30 percent or more. For delivery, C-section is appropriate if there is bleeding and pregnancy greater than 35 weeks with confirmed fetal lung maturity and previa, fetal distress, and increased hemorrhage. A vaginal delivery may be appropriate if the placenta is low lying and a viable fetus is in cephalic presentation, or if there is a nonviable fetus in which there may be a greater degree of previa.

## VASA PREVIA

*Vasa previa* occurs when the fetal umbilical cord vessels pass over the internal cervical os preceding the fetal presenting part. Ultrasound imaging usually is not able to identify the vessels and this condition is also characterized by *painless bleeding*. This is a very rare occurrence and is usually associated with vilamentous cord insertions and/or multiple gestations. The classic *triad* of vasa previa is: (1) *rupture of membranes*, (2) *bleeding*, and (3) *fetal bradycardia*. The greatest risk of fetal hemorrhage or exsanguination is at the time of *membrane rupture*. The fetal vessels cross membranes that are overlying the internal cervical os, and when the membranes rupture, this causes tearing of the vessels. The only management is immediate *delivery*.

## UTERINE RUPTURE

*Uterine rupture* is characterized by *painful bleeding*, and is a full thickness laceration of the myometrial wall. There are *four* types of uterine rupture:

### Incomplete rupture
The incomplete rupture has the peritoneal cavity separated from the uterine cavity by the visceral peritoneum.

### Complete rupture
This has a laceration that communicates directly with the peritoneal cavity, and is divided into spontaneous and traumatic sub-types.

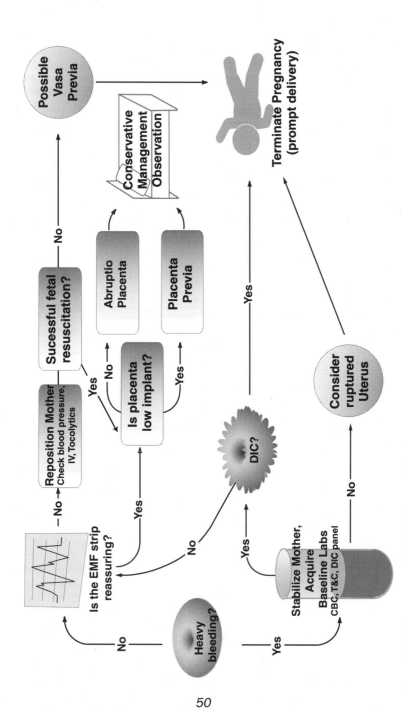

**Figure 4-5** Management of Third Trimester Bleeding.

### C-section scar rupture
The old incision separates throughout most of its length with all or part of fetal extrusion into the peritoneal cavity, with massive bleeding, 50 percent fetal death, and 5 percent maternal death occurring.

### Dehiscence
This is the gradual and asymptomatic separation of only *part of* the old C-section incision—usually these are considered to be *incomplete ruptures.*

Uterine rupture occurs in 1 in 1500 deliveries and may be associated with previous classical uterine incision, overuse of oxytocin, grand multiparity, marked uterine distention, and external or internal version. Most of the complications are associated with causes of bleeding and immediate delivery. They include: hemorrhage, shock, post operative infection, urethral damage, thrombophlebitis, amniotic fluid embolism, DIC, pituitary failure, future infertility, and death. In rupture, prevention is the key; therefore, estimated fetal weight, supervised oxytocin administration, and good closure of C-section incisions are all important. Otherwise, treatment includes antibiotics, rupture repair if childbearing is an issue, ipsilateral hypogastric artery ligation for hemostasis if lower uterine segment is involved, and if complete rupture is the case then a hysterectomy (Fig. 4-5).

## ECTOPIC PREGNANCY

An *ectopic pregnancy* occurs when the fertilized ovum is implanted *outside of* the endometrial cavity. It presents as a triad of: abdominal *pain*, vaginal *bleeding*, and *amenorrhea*. Furthermore, the patient will likely be afebrile, and have *abdominal tenderness* and an *adnexal mass* on examination. Ectopic pregnancy occurs in 1 in 100 pregnancies with a maternal mortality rate of 1 to 2 percent. Over 75 percent are diagnosed before 12 weeks of gestation, and 40 percent of these pregnancies occur in females between the ages of 20 and 29. Usually these young females have a history of *multiple partners*, IUD use, PID, and STDs. Ten to twenty percent of the women have recurrent ectopics with 4 to 5 percent occurring in the opposite tube. Consider a *threatened abortion* in these patients. Fifty percent of women will have a normal pregnancy after an ectopic, but another 50 percent will develop infertility problems after surgery and of these, 30 percent will be sterile. Symptoms of an *acutely ruptured* ectopic pregnancy include: increased abdominal pain and distention, possible shoulder pain, and *hypovolemia* (check for compensation, like increased heart rate).

Treatment is *salpingostomy.* You should perform an ultrasound and consider culdocentesis (aspiration of rectouterine peritoneal fluid *transvaginally* to check for blood in the cul-de-sac), laparoscopy under general anesthesia, and laparotomy in the *Trendelenberg position* (angle the patient so that the head is lowered and the feet are up—this allows the bowels to go *down*, away from the area of surgery).

There are *five different types* of ectopic pregnancy—based on their location:

### TUBAL ECTOPICS

These account for more than 99 percent of ectopics, and can be subdivided into *ampullary* (55 percent), *isthmic* (25 percent), fimbrial (17 percent), interstitial (angular or cornual, 2 percent), and bilateral. Remember, a common location for ectopic pregnancy is at the *ampulla* of the *fallopian tube*. Tubal pregnancies may terminate by abortion, missed abortion, or rupture. Isthmic, ruptures often occur at 6 to 8 weeks, ampullary at 8 to 12 weeks, and interstitial at 16 to 20 weeks. Angular ectopics may be carried to *term* since the nidation point is just inside the uterine cavity. This type is potentially lethal and may often require a hysterectomy as an emergency procedure.

Interstitial, angular, and cornual pregnancies may *rupture* into the *uterine cavity* or *uterine wall*—which may divide, causing severe local destruction of the myometrium; or they may *rupture* into the *broad ligament* or directly into the *peritoneal cavity*.

### OVARIAN ECTOPICS

These account for less than 0.5 percent of ectopics, and may follow the fertilization of an unextruded ovum. These almost never reach viability and usually rupture into the peritoneal cavity, but may also dissect into the folds of the ovarian ligament or form a *lithopedion*.

### ABDOMINAL ECTOPICS

These pregnancies occur in about 1 in 15,000 or less than 0.1 percent of ectopics. The pregnancy may be considered *primary* if the initial implantation of the zygote occurs outside of the tube or *secondary* if the zygote is released via rupture or expulsion. These may rupture into the peritoneal cavity, retroperitoneal space, or into a vital organ. Also, they may form a mass called an *adipocere* or a *lithopedion*, which is an *intraperitoneal abscess* from infected fetal parts. Pregnancies of this type may continue to an advanced stage.

### CERVICAL ECTOPICS

If a greatly enlarged cervix known as an "hourglass sign" (a very rare occurrence) is noted then a cervical ectopic should be expected. These may grow to be as large as the non-pregnant uterus and are characterized by a highly vascularized, bleeding cervix with a tight internal os and a gaping external os. An ectopic of this type may be complicated by *rupture* into the *cervical canal* and move directly into the *vagina*, and rarely, into the base of the *broad ligament* with the complication of an intra-abdominal hematoma.

### COMBINED OR HETEROTOPIC PREGNANCY

This occurs in about 1 in 17,000 to 30,000 ectopics, and is the combination of a *tubal* and an *intrauterine pregnancy*. The most common complaints are abdominal and pelvic *pain*, abnormal uterine *bleeding*, and *amenorrhea*. Complications include: *maternal death* in 1 in 1000 ectopic cases, *hemorrhage*, chronic salpingitis, infertility or sterility, intestinal obstruction, hemoperitoneum, fistula, and peritonitis. The management includes: surgery by *laparotomy* or *laparoscopy*—depending on if the patient is hemodynamically stable in the cases of *rupture*. If she has NOT ruptured, and the pregnancy is early on, then you may treat with *methotrexate* and follow the quantitative β-hCG levels every 48 h. If there are signs of *infection*, then a broad-spectrum antibiotic is indicated.

## PREMATURE LABOR

Labor occurring *after* **20** weeks but *before* **36** weeks is defined as *premature* labor. Clinical signs include: *contractions* that occur every 5 min (for at least half an hour), and evidence of *cervical change*—either *effacement* or *dilatation* or both. There should NOT be any rupture of membranes and NO evidence of abruption or previa. Premature labor occurs in about 5 to 15 percent of all pregnancies. Some of the most common risk factors include: pre-eclampsia, placental insufficiency, multiple gestation, polyhydramnios, abnormal placentation, tobacco, drug, or alcohol use, infection, uterine anomalies, previous premature birth, trauma, and previous uterine incision—just to name a few. It is very important to rule out any infectious causes, electrolyte abnormalities, and chorioamnionitis. An **L/S** (Lecithin/**S**phingomyelin) *ratio* will assess the lung *maturity*. The normal L/S ratio is >2, and there is an increased chance for *respiratory distress syndrome* if the L/S ratio is <2.

The management includes: tocolysis with *β-2 adrenergic agonists* (such as terbutaline, ritodrine, or isoxsuprine)—which all act to *relax* smooth muscle; *magnesium sulfate*—which competes with calcium during depolarization to help relax smooth muscle; or with the new trial agents such as *prostaglandin inhibitors* (like indomethacin and aspirin), and *calcium-channel blockers* (like nifedipine). It is also important to supply IV fluids for hydration and glucocorticoids (such as betamethasone) to help decrease the incidence of acute respiratory distress in the prematurely born neonate.

## PREMATURE RUPTURE OF MEMBRANES (PROM)

If rupture of membranes occurs *greater than* 24 h before the onset of labor, whether the fetus is considered premature or mature, it is defined as *premature rupture of membranes*. The incidence in all pregnancies is around 11 percent with 94 percent of the cases in mature fetuses, 20 percent complicated by prolonged rupture, and with 5 percent of the cases in premature fetuses, 50 percent complicated by prolonged rupture. This is more commonly associated with maternal infection, intrauterine infection, cervical incompetence, **multi**parity, polyhydramnios, nutritional defects, and previous history of premature rupture.

The evaluation for a patient with complaints of premature rupture might include: a sterile speculum exam (for positive pooling, *ferning*, and nitrazine), cultures from the cervix and the fluid (for signs of infection), fluid evaluation (for L/S ratio), ultrasound (for amniotic fluid volume), and other lab tests (to rule out infection—tests such as CBC with differential, and urine culture and sensitivity).

Management in most cases would involve *delivery*. If the infant is *premature* and there is time, *betamethasone* may be given to *decrease* neonatal respiratory distress, and then deliver the baby. If the fetus is *less than* **26** weeks, then there is little chance of survival and pregnancy *termination* may be considered.

---

## POST-DATES

Post-dates are defined as pregnancies that have reached **42** weeks from the first day of the last menstrual period (LMP), and occur in approximately 3 percent of pregnancies. Risk factors include: *lack of* normally high levels of estrogen, anencephaly, fetal adrenal hypoplasia, fetal pituitary absence, placental sulfatase insufficiency, and extra-uterine (abdominal) pregnancy. *Delivery* will be by induction or if necessary by C-section if indicated for the management of these cases. Complications may include: fetal macrosomia, aging or infected placenta, shoulder dystocia, oligohydramnios, and cord compromise.

---

## INAPPROPRIATE FETAL GROWTH

### SMALL FOR GESTATIONAL AGE

Small for gestational age (SGA) and intrauterine growth restriction (IUGR) are defined as fetuses that score less than the *tenth* percentile for fetal growth. There are two types described—symmetric and asymmetric.

*Symmetric* has a normal amniotic fluid volume and accounts for about 20 percent of the cases. It shows a *symmetric* decrease in all body parts such as that seen on ultrasound in the biparietal diameter, head circumference, abdominal circumference, and femur length. Usually it is caused by an early pregnancy insult and/or a fetal problem such as cytogenetic, infectious, or anomalies. Cytogenetic causes can be *autosomal,* such as trisomy 13, 18, 21, and *chromosomal deletions*, sex chromosomal problems such as Turner's and multiple chromosomes, neural tube defects, and dysmorphic syndromes such as achondroplasia and osteogenesis imperfecta.

Infections that can be associated with *symmetric* IUGR include: viral infections seen in "TORCH" such as toxoplasmosis, rubella, CMV, HSV, and VZV as well as protozoan, malarial, and bacterial infections (like listeriosis). Important drugs to consider are: alcohol, tobacco, warfarin, and folic acid antagonists (such as methotrexate and aminopterin), and anticonvulsants and radiation also may be associated.

*Asymmetric* IUGR occurs in about 80 percent of the cases and shows a brain-sparing effect on ultrasound—meaning there is a *decrease* in abdominal circumference and a *decrease* in amniotic fluid volume, with the other parameters normal. This is usually from a late pregnancy *insult* and usually placenta-mediated—such as problems with maternal hypertension, poor nutrition, and smoking. Also, there may be some relation to *multiple gestations, maternal disorders* such as renal disease, pancreatitis, intestinal parasites, and anemia, as well as placental disorders such as placenta previa, placenta malformations, chorionic villitis, and chorionic partial separation. *Prevention* is the key in all cases of IUGR, either through genetic screening or maternal avoidance of external factors. If fetal-maternal monitoring reveals fetal compromise, then you may want to consider delivery. The most common complications include: fetal *hypoxia* and acidosis, fetal *malformation*, *stillbirth*, neonatal hypoglycemia, neonatal meconium aspiration syndrome, SIDS, lower IQ, learning and behavioral problems, seizure disorders, cerebral palsy, and severe mental retardation.

## LARGE FOR GESTATIONAL AGE

Large for gestational age (LGA) fetuses have a growth curve with fetal growth *greater than* **90 percent**. Risk factors include: maternal disorders such as *diabetes*, *obesity*, **multi**parity, advanced maternal *age*, previous *history* of large infant, large stature, post-dates, and *fetal disorders* such as male sex, and genetic or *congenital disorders* such as *Beckwith-Wiedemann Syndrome* (pancreatic islet cell hyperplasia, macroglossia), Weaver's, Soto's, Nevo, and fragile X syndromes.

Best management is *delivery earlier* than the EDC, either by labor induction or C-section if indicated. Complications include: maternal operative delivery via C-section or operative vaginal delivery, maternal postpartum *hemorrhage*, and perineal trauma. Fetal and neonatal complications include: low APGARS, hypoglycemia, shoulder dystocia, birth injury, hypocalcemia, polycythemia, jaundice, feeding difficulties, stillbirth, and anomalies. Some long-term complications include: *obesity*, type II *diabetes*, neuro-behavioral problems, and childhood onset of cancer.

## MULTIPLE GESTATIONS

Multiple gestation is defined as the demonstration of *two or more* fetuses *in utero*. Incidence of *twins* is 1 in 80, while the incidence of *triplets* is 1 in 6400, and the incidence of *quadruplets* decreases to 1 in 512,000. Complications incurred may be twin-to-twin transfusion syndrome, villamentous cord insertion, two-vessel cord, or monochorionic, monoamnionic twins leading to cord entanglement. Furthermore, the average age of gestation is 35 weeks (versus 39). There are two types of twins, *monozygotic* and *dizygotic* (Fig. 4-6).

### MONOZYGOTIC TWINS

These twins (approximately ⅓ of all twins) result from fertilization of a *single ovum* by a *single sperm* that gives *maternal* or "identical" twins. If division occurs *prior to* the morula stage and differentiation of the trophoblast, then (as occurs in *one-third* of the cases) there will be separate or fused placentas, two chorions, and two amnions. If division occurs *after* differentiation of the trophoblast, but before the formation of the amnion, then there will be one placenta, a common chorion, and two amnions—seen in *two-thirds* of monozygotic cases. If division occurs *after* differentiation of the *amnion*, then there will be one placenta, one chorion, and *one* amnion—but this is rare. If the division occurs later than the 14th day, then this may result in *incomplete twinning*. If it is between the 8th and the 14th day, this may result in *conjoined twins*.

# Dizygotic Twins

## Nonidentical or Fraternal Twins
**(Always have 2 chorions and 2 amnions,
and sexes may be different.)**

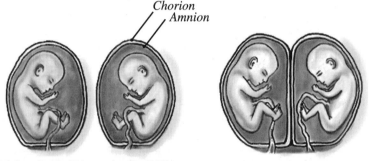

*Chorion*
*Amnion*

**Dichorionic Diamnionic (1/3)**
*separate development*

**Dichorionic Diamnionic (1/3)**
*fused development*

# Monozygotic Twins
## Identical or Maternal Twins

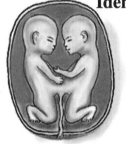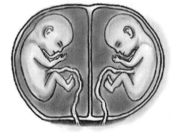

**Monochorionic
Monoamnionic (rare)**
*(Siamese twins)*
*Twins share single cavity*

**Monochorionic
Diamnionic (<1/3)**
*Twins are in separate cavities*

**Figure 4-6**   Twin Placentas.

### DIZYGOTIC TWINS

These twins (approximately ⅔ of all twins) result from the product of *two ovum* and *two sperms* that give *fraternal* or non-identical twins. If division occurs *prior to* the morula stage and differentiation of the trophoblast, then (as occurs in *most* of the cases) there will be separate or fused placentas, two chorions and two amnions.

---

## OLIGOHYDRAMNIOS

This is defined as a marked *deficiency* in the volume of amniotic fluid. This may be due to umbilical *cord compression* or *spontaneous ROM*.

---

## POLYHYDRAMNIOS

This is defined as excessive amounts of amniotic fluid (greater than 2 liters). Twins have an increased risk of premature labor.
Fetal anomalies: Respiratory or Gastrointestinal.

---

## ISOIMMUNIZATION

In Rh isoimmunization, if an Rh-*negative* mother has an Rh-*positive* fetus, and the mother has a history of previous exposure or a *previous* infant with **hemolytic disease of the newborn**, then isoimmunization may be encountered. Hemolytic disease of the newborn is when the *maternal* antibodies destroy Rh-*positive* fetal red blood cells, causing fetal *anemia*, with the complication of **fetal hydrops** and stillbirth.

*Rhogam,* or anti-D γ-globulin (IgG), is given to *all* Rh-*negative* mothers (the mother *lacks* the Rh antigen on the red blood cell). Furthermore, it is especially given if the father is Rh positive or the baby is Rh positive. A titration is necessary, and Rhogam should be given within the first 72 h after delivery, and it should be given at 28 weeks gestation in mothers who are Rh negative. The *Kleihauer-Betke test* is used to get an estimate of the extent of fetal to maternal hemorrhage by removing the *adult* hemoglobin, and *staining* the *fetal* cells to count the number of *fetal cells* divided by the number of *maternal cells.*

ABO incompatibilities are much milder than Rh incompatibilities and almost always associated with group A or B infants of group O mothers (with complications of stillbirth, fetal anemia, and fetal hydrops almost NEVER occurring). The most common complication is *early neonatal jaundice.*

---

## HYPEREMESIS GRAVIDARUM

This is intractable nausea and *vomiting* during pregnancy that may require hospitalization due to severe *dehydration* and *ketonuria*. This may be due to rapidly rising levels of hCG (as high as 100,000 mU/ml in the first trimester). This can be managed by a dry, bland, light diet, eating smaller portions and more frequent meals, and emotional support if it is uncomplicated. If the symptoms are more severe, then the mother may need IV fluid hydration, possible TPN, and hospitalization with the use of IV drugs such as phenergan, compazine, tigan, reglan, and thorazine as a last resort. This may be associated more frequently with molar pregnancies.

## PREGNANCY-INDUCED HYPERTENSION (PREECLAMPSIA)

This is defined as an elevated blood pressure of **30** mmHg systolic and **15** mmHg diastolic above the baseline blood pressure, proteinuria defined as >300 mg of protein in a 24-h urine specimen, and edema. It occurs in about 6 percent of the general population and presents during the late second or after the second trimester. NOTE: If it occurs prior to the second trimester, then consider a *hydatidiform mole* or *chronic hypertension* as possibilities. Risk factors include: nulliparity, black race, maternal age <20 or >35, low socio-economic status, multiple gestation, hydatidiform mole, polyhydramnios, non-immune fetal hydrops, diabetes, chronic hypertension, and renal disease. There are two categories defined, *mild* and *severe*. *Severe* is defined by persistent *proteinuria* of 2+ or more or >4 g in a 24-h urine sample. Mild and severe pre-eclampsia are differentiated by:

1. BP > 160 mmHg systolic and > 110 mmHg diastolic
2. *Proteinuria* > 5 g in 24-h urine or 3 to 4+ on urine dipstick
3. Increase in serum *creatinine* > 1.2 mg/dl (unless already increased pre-pregnancy)
4. Cerebral or visual disturbances
5. Epigastric pain
6. Increased liver enzymes
7. Thrombocytopenia with <100,000 mm$^3$ of platelets
8. Retinal hemorrhages, exudates, and papilledema
9. Pulmonary edema

The **HELLP syndrome** is a derivative of PIH that consists of: *hemolysis, elevated liver enzymes*, and *low platelet count*. Furthermore, there may or may not be an elevated blood pressure. Usually it occurs in a **multi**parous woman over 25 years of age, and in a pregnancy *less* than 36 weeks.

Management includes: the use of blood pressure lowering agents (such as aldomet or a calcium-channel blocker, and bed rest in the *left lateral* position in *mild* cases; and *hydralazine*, methyldopa, and magnesium sulfate in *severe* cases). The only sure cure of the problem is *delivery* of the infant (especially if >36 weeks gestation). Remember, *eclampsia* is defined by maternal *convulsions* due to an *elevated blood pressure*.

## Types of Hypertensive Disorders in Pregnancy

| | Mild PIH | Serve PIH | Eclampsia | Chronic HTN | Chronic HTN/ PIH | Transient HTN |
|---|---|---|---|---|---|---|
| **Blood Pressure** | ≥140/90 ↑15 diast. and/ or ↑30 syst. | ≥160/110 | AlmPIH | HTN<20 wks or pre-existing HTN | >baseline | AlmPIH |
| **Proteinuria** | 1-2 + dipstick or >o.3gm/ day | 3-4+ dipstick or >5gm/ day | AlmPIH | None to Variable | AlmPIH, or >baseline | Ø |
| **Edema in Extremities** | Variable | Variable | Variable | None to Variable | None to Variable | Ø |
| **Convulsions** | Ø | Ø | **YES** | Ø | Ø | Ø |
| **Symptoms: HA epigastric pain, other changes** | Ø | Maybe | Maybe | Ø | Maybe | Ø |
| **DIC: ↓platelets ↓Fibrinogen,↑PTT ↑PT** | Ø | Maybe | Maybe | Ø | Maybe | Ø |
| **Cyanosis, Pulmonary edema** | Ø | Maybe | Maybe | Variable | Ø | Ø |

AlmPIH = At least mild PIH criteria
Ø = none

**Figure 4-7**   Types of Hypertensive Disorders in Pregnancy

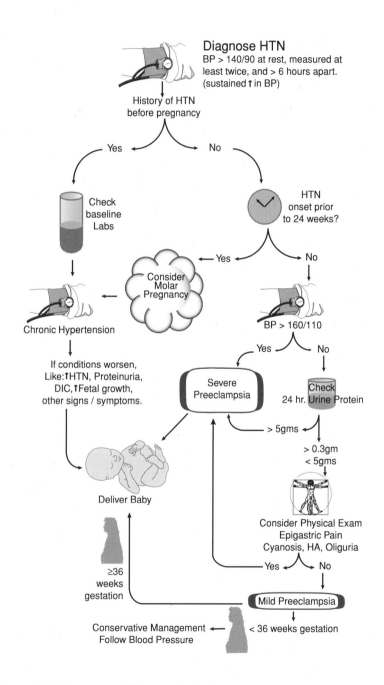

**Diagnose HTN**
BP > 140/90 at rest, measured at least twice, and > 6 hours apart. (sustained ↑ in BP)

History of HTN before pregnancy

Yes

No

Check baseline Labs

HTN onset prior to 24 weeks?

Yes

No

Consider Molar Pregnancy

Chronic Hypertension

BP > 160/110

If conditions worsen, Like:↑HTN, Proteinuria, DIC,↑Fetal growth, other signs / symptoms.

Yes

No

Severe Preeclampsia

Check 24 hr. Urine Protein

> 5gms

> 0.3gm
< 5gms

Deliver Baby

Consider Physical Exam
Epigastric Pain
Cyanosis, HA, Oliguria

Yes

No

≥36 weeks gestation

Mild Preeclampsia

< 36 weeks gestation

Conservative Management
Follow Blood Pressure

**Figure 4-8**  Management of Hypertension in Pregnancy

## GESTATIONAL DIABETES MELLITUS

This is a chronic condition during pregnancy that affects the metabolism of carbohydrates, proteins, and fats. There is a classification of diabetes called the *White classification* of diabetes in pregnancy. Class **A** refers to *gestational diabetes* with the onset *in* pregnancy. (Try to remember Class $A_1$, which is developed during pregnancy and has a relatively *normal* fasting blood glucose—the treatment is *dietary control*. Class $A_2$ is controlled by *diet* and *insulin*, since these patients have elevated fasting glucose.) Class **B** is the onset of diabetes *after age 20*, with a duration of less than 10 years and NO vascular disease. Class **C** is an onset between ages *10 and 19* years, with a duration of 10 to 19 years and NO vascular disease. Class **D** is the onset *before* age 10, with a duration of greater than 20 years and some vascular disease (such as retinopathy or peripheral vascular disease). Class **E** includes *pelvic arteriosclerosis* (seen on x-ray). Class **F** is associated with *vascular nephritis*. Class **R** refers to *proliferative retinopathy* and class **T** refers to transplantation. Usually, if diabetes is not diagnosed prior to pregnancy, then most pregnant women are diagnosed during their routine glucose screening at 24 to 28 weeks with a 50 g glucose load and checking the serum glucose level 1 h later. If the serum glucose is >135 mg/dl then it is considered a *positive screen* and the woman has a 3-h glucose tolerance test where she is given a 100 g glucose load and the values are evaluated at time 0, 1, 2, and 3 h after ingestion.

Blood glucose levels should be <90, <165, <145, and <125 for the respective hours above for the test to be considered negative. Maternal complications include hypoglycemia and hyperglycemia, insulin shifts, glucosuria, urinary tract infections, hypertension, hydramnios, and retinopathy. After delivery, usually the insulin requirement is *decreased* to *none*, and you need to check the glucose level every 6 h—if the glucose is greater than **150**, consider giving *insulin*.

Fetal problems include: spontaneous abortion, congenital anomalies such as sacral agenesis and limb deformities, macrosomia, neonatal hypoglycemia, respiratory difficulties, perinatal death, and other problems such as hypocalcemia, hyperbilirubinemia, polycythemia, and renal vein thrombosis. Management includes adequate diet control, close glucose monitoring, insulin as indicated, routine ultrasounds to assess fetal growth and development and fetal well-being, and ophthalmologic examination.

# *Reproductive Contraception and Sterilization*

5

---

## *TYPES OF CONTRACEPTION*

### NATURAL FAMILY PLANNING

Natural family planning refers to the use of *timed abstention* from sexual intercourse in order to avoid the most fertile times of the menstrual cycle. *This has lower* success rates than barrier methods, intrauterine methods, or steroid contraceptives, due to difficulty in predicting ovulation, and it requires prolonged abstinence of up to 17 days per cycle. Timing is done through calendar-based methods such as the **rhythm method,** also called the *periodic abstinence method,* which follows the predictable occurrence of ovulation, or *planned intercourse* based on the *basal body temperature* and *cervical mucus monitoring.*

### BARRIER CONTRACEPTIVES

These can be divided into the *five* different types listed below.

#### Condoms

Condoms are divided into male and female types. The *male version* is a latex condom that is applied to the penis. The latex is effective up to 1 to 5/100 woman years for preventing pregnancy and is also more effective than other contraceptives in preventing the transmission of HIV and other STDs; however, condoms are not completely fail-proof. The *female version* is a vaginal pouch made of polyurethane or latex that covers a portion of the vulva as well and acts as a barrier.

#### Diaphragms

A diaphragm is a *barrier method* that comes in three styles, called **coil, flat**, and **arching spring** (which is the most commonly used type). They also range in size from 50 to 105 mm. Diaphragms should be big enough to *cover the entire cervix* and almost the entire anterior surface of the vagina. Failure rates may range from 2 to 15 failures per 100 woman-years. The three most important principles of diaphragm use are proper positioning, inserting fresh spermicide in the vagina, and leaving the diaphragm in place for a sufficient period of time following intercourse, usually for six or more hours. Diaphragm users are about twice as likely to experience urinary tract symptoms than users of oral contraceptives.

### Spermicides
Spermicides are another form of *barrier contraceptive* that can be purchased over the counter (like condoms)—whereas diaphragms must be fitted and prescribed by a physician. They come in creams, jellies, foams, films, and suppositories. Nonoxynol-9 is the most commonly used spermicide in the United States today. These can either be used alone if the concentration is high enough, 3 to 20% nonoxynol-9, but may cause more vaginal and penile *irritation*, or may be used at a lower concentration in conjunction with another barrier method such as the diaphragm, condom, or cervical cap. The effectiveness of spermicides demands compliance and proper usage; the spermicide must be used with every episode of sexual intercourse and new spermicide should be reapplied if the previous dose has been left in the vagina for more than 1 h.

### Vaginal sponges
A vaginal sponge is a polyurethane, dimpled *disk* that contains the *spermicide* nonoxynol-9 and is placed in the vagina over the cervix for up to 24 h prior to coitus. It may remain in the vagina for up to 24 h after coitus, but cannot exceed a total time in the vagina of 30 h.

### Cervical caps
Cervical caps have shown in trials to be as effective as the diaphragm, although they are somewhat harder to fit and to insert. As with the diaphragm, these must be left in place for at least 6 h after intercourse, but they may be left in place up to several days without any increased risk of toxic shock syndrome, but this should not be done during menses.

### INTRAUTERINE DEVICES OR IUDS
IUDs offer highly effective, long-lasting, inexpensive, and completely reversible contraceptive protection. But, if infection occurs, this device does *not* offer "reversible" protection. These work by preventing fertilization of the ovum by interfering with tubal function and sperm function. There are two types used today, the *Progestasert* and the *Paragard.*

The Progestasert is a *hormonal* IUD that contains 36mg of progesterone that produces local changes in the endometrium and the cervical mucus. This type must be replaced every twelve months due to the progesterone only being released for 15 to 24 months, and has a higher ectopic and total pregnancy rate than the copper IUDs.

The Paragard consists of a plastic *stem* bearing tightly wound copper wire and arms with *copper sheaths*. It provides highly effective contraception for up to eight years by interfering with the events of fertilization and possibly implantation. IUDs are inserted into the *endometrial cavity.* In addition to preventing fertilization, they may also act by *inhibiting implantation* and changing the *motility* and *endometrium*.

In general, IUDs are *absolutely contraindicated* in known or suspected pregnancy, undiagnosed vaginal bleeding, previous PID, and known or suspected pelvic malignancy (cancer). Furthermore, IUDs are *relatively contraindicated* in sexual practices that increase the risk of contracting STDs, nulliparity (because of the risk of *pelvic infection* and *infertility*), unresolved abnormal Pap smears, uterine anomalies of shape or size, and medical conditions that may increase the risk of infections such as diabetes. IUDs should be reserved for *multiparous* women who cannot take oral contraceptives (woman smoking in her 30s).

Complications include: PID, ectopic pregnancy, spontaneous abortion, and altered menses. IUDs have a low failure rate (5 percent in the first year, and only 1 to 2 percent after the first year). IUD users have a four to five times increased risk of developing an *ectopic* if *pregnancy* occurs, a higher risk of *salpingo-oophoritis*, *abscess*, *pelvic infection* (especially young, nulliparous women), a subclinical risk of *endometriosis*, and *infertility*. In a patient who has conceived, there is an increased risk of *abortion*.

## STEROID ORAL CONTRACEPTIVES

These most commonly contain two different synthetic derivatives of naturally occurring *estradiol* (an estrogen) and *19-nortestosterone* (a progestin). Most of the OCPs contain 30 to 35 µg of ethinyl estradiol and the progestin can vary from 0.15 to 1 mg of several varying types of progestin. The dosing pattern can either be fixed with a fixed ratio of progestin to estrogen throughout the pill cycle or phased with a varying ratio of progestin to estrogen over the cycle.

OCPs act by *inhibiting gonadotropin secretion* by action on the hypothalamus and the pituitary, and by creating an unfavorable *endometrial lining* that resists implantation through the progesterone effect.

They are *contraindicated* in: existing thrombophlebitis, thromboembolic disorders, cerebral vascular or coronary artery disease, breast carcinoma, estrogen-dependent neoplasia, undiagnosed abnormal vaginal bleeding, pregnancy, and active liver disease. Side effects include: headaches, acne, nausea, breast soreness, hair loss, and increased skin pigmentation.

*Risks* of oral contraceptive use include thromboembolism, CVA and hypertension (in smokers), amenorrhea, cholelithiasis, and hepatic tumors. (Developing breast cancer is NOT considered a risk.)

## PROGESTIN-ONLY CONTRACEPTIVES

These are divided into *oral, injectable,* and *implantable contraceptives.* The **oral pills** or "mini-pills" act by the use of adequate doses of progestin to suppress ovulation and to inhibit fertility by altering cervical mucus and the endometrium. This form of contraception is particularly useful in women with contraindications to the estrogen in combined OCPs. **Depo-Provera** is an *intramuscular injection* that acts over three months to prevent pregnancy under the same principle as the oral progestins. The side effects are also similar, but the patient is more likely to experience amenorrhea after a series of every-three-month injections and normal return of ovulation may be delayed up to one year after discontinuation. **Norplant** is a long-term *implantable progestin* that provides contraception for up to five years. Six silastic *tubes* are placed in the upper arm under the skin, and act by providing low levels of progestin continually, providing effective contraception. This form does require a procedure performed by the physician under sterile conditions for insertion and removal. For both norplant and depo-provera, there is a slightly increased complaint of *weight gain* while using these forms of birth control.

## POST-COITAL CONTRACEPTION

This works by giving a *high* dose of estrogen promptly after intercourse to prevent fertilization. Most commonly a combined OCP containing 50 μg of ethinyl estradiol and 0.5 mg of norgestrel is used within 72 h of intercourse to be effective. Two tablets are given immediately and then again 12 h later. Common side effects include: nausea, breast soreness, and, less commonly, thrombotic effects. Also, copper IUDs can be used in this way if inserted within three days of unprotected intercourse.

## STERILIZATION AND ELECTIVE PREGNANCY TERMINATION

Female sterilization most often involves operative interruption of the fallopian tubes and may either be done by laparotomy during the first 24 to 48 h postpartum or as an interval procedure at any time while not pregnant, by laparotomy, minilap, laparoscopy, or culpotomy. Hysterectomy may also be used for sterilization purposes if uterine disease is present. Male sterilization involves doing a procedure called a vasectomy. Informed consent is an important part of the preoperative counseling process. Candidates for sterilization must understand that the procedure is *meant to be permanent* and understand the *risks of failure,* including ectopic pregnancy and the risk of intraoperative and postoperative complications. *Tubal ligation* is contraindicated in pregnancy, and cardiovascular or pulmonary disease, and may be also contraindicated in women with a history of major intra-abdominal surgery or severe PID or endometriosis. Postoperative complications may immediately include hemorrhage and infection and, later on, pregnancy occurring in 0.2 to 0.8 percent. The most serious problem is the risk of *ectopic pregnancy*, which is highest among women who have had unipolar electrocoagulation procedures and lowest among those having the Pomeroy for postpartum tubals, the clip, or Silastic ring procedures.

An *elective or induced abortion* is a procedure intended to terminate an intrauterine pregnancy prior to viability. Often these procedures are performed to treat or prevent medical complications of pregnancy. One of every four pregnancies is electively aborted. Maternal morbidity and mortality increases with advancing gestation and there is a higher risk associated with general anesthesia versus local anesthesia. The legal statistics regarding abortion rights of women can be divided into thirds: with ⅓ of the world's women living in societies with nonrestrictive laws dealing with abortion, ⅓ living in societies with some legal restrictions concerning abortions, and ⅓ living where abortion is considered illegal. Refer to the following table for methods of abortion, their procedure type, and risks and complications involved (Table 5-1.)

| Induced Abortion | | | | | |
|---|---|---|---|---|---|
| | Weeks Gestation (after missed period) | Method | Anesthesia | Risks/ Complications | Mortality Rate |
| **Menstrual extraction** | <2 | *Syringe* aspiration | None | Failure of termination | 0 |
| **Suction curettage** | <12 weeks | *Vacuum* aspiration | Local/ Sedatives | Bleeding, Infection, Perforated uterus | 1/100,000 |
| **Sharp curettage** | <12 weeks | *Sharp scraping* | Local/ Sedatives | Bleeding, Infection, Perforated uterus, A Sherman's Syndrome | 1/100,000 |
| **Dilation & Evacuation** | 14–20 weeks | *Morcellation* (Dividing fetus into small parts & removal) | Paracervical block/ Sedatives | Bleeding, Infection Cervical laceration, Perforated uterus | 4/100,000 |
| **Amnionic infusion/ Vaginal suppository** | ≥14 weeks | Induce labor by contractions; $PGF_{2\alpha}$ or $PGE_2$, Hypertonic saline, Hyperosm. urea | Blocks/ Narcotics | Bleeding, Cervical laceration, Retained placenta | 8/100,000 |
| **Hysterotomy/ Hysterectomy** | Any age during gestation | Minor C-section removing the uterus (with fetus) | General | Bleeding, Infection, Visceral injury | 25/100,000 |

# The Menstrual Cycle and Disorders of Menstruation

# 6

---

## THE MENSTRUAL CYCLE

The menstrual cycle refers to the repetitive, ovulation-mediated occurrence of uterine bleeding typically occurring every 28 days. The most common range is 26 to 30 days, but the cycle can range from 24 to 40 days in length. The average duration of flow is 5 days, but may range from 3 to 7 days; the average blood loss is only about 40 ml. The *two phases* of the menstrual cycle are the *follicular phase* and the *luteal phase*. (A third phase could be considered the *menstrual phase*.)

The **follicular phase** coincides with the time of ovarian follicular growth that precedes ovulation and is also known as the *proliferative phase (estrogenic phase)*—which reflects the pattern of endometrial development during this time (see Fig. 6-1). This phase is mediated by follicular responses to follicle-stimulating hormone and its varying length is responsible for the differences in the length of the menstrual cycle. Its onset is the *first day* of menses, and it ceases the day of *ovulation*. The basal body temperature is low and estrogen is the dominant hormone with increased production at day 13 to 14, and LH and FSH will spike around day 15. The uterine lining is thin and the glands are drawn out and lengthening. Luteinizing hormone and follicle-stimulating hormone are mediated by GnRH, (gonadotropin-releasing hormone), which is synthesized in the hypothalamus and secreted into the hypophyseal-portal circulation. This stimulates the release of FSH and LH from the anterior portion of the pituitary gland.

The role of LH and FSH is to stimulate *both gonadal production* of sex steroids and *ovum maturation*. FSH receptors are found in the granulosa cells of the ovary and when FSH binds it stimulates the formation of LH receptors, enzymes aromatase, and 3-hydroxysteroid dehydrogenase, which are responsible for the production of estrogen. LH receptors are found in the theca cells, granulosa cells, and the corpus luteum of the ovary. The primary action of LH on the ovary is the *stimulation of androgen production* by the theca cells and *progesterone synthesis* by the corpus luteum.

The **luteal phase** or the *postovulatory phase* is characterized by development of an edematous, glycogen-secreting endometrial lining and progesterone secretion (see Fig. 6-1). This phase is also called the *secretory phase* (progestational phase) due to the effect on the endometrium. The length is

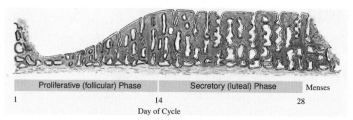

**Figure 6-1**  Endometrium during the menstrual cycle.

constant at a range of 12 to 16 days with the onset on the day of ovulation and the termination at the onset of menses. The basal body temperature is increased here. Progesterone is the dominant hormone with a spike at 21 to 23 days and the uterine lining is thick with thick and tortuous glands (Fig. 6-1).

As the corpus luteum regresses and progesterone decreases, the endometrium "sloughs off." This is the menstrual phase (menses).

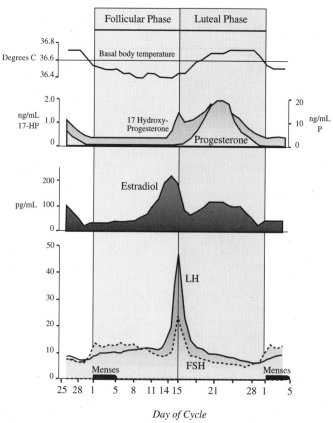

**Figure 6-2**  The Menstrual Cycle

---

## DISORDERS OF MENSTRUATION

### AMENORRHEA

This refers to the *complete absence* of vaginal bleeding in the reproductive-age woman and is considered a symptom, not a diagnosis. The absence of menstruation is considered to be normal and physiologic prior to puberty, during pregnancy and lactation, and after menopause. Amenorrhea is divided into two types, called *primary* amenorrhea and *secondary* amenorrhea.

#### Primary amenorrhea

This refers to females who fail to undergo menarche or development of secondary sexual characteristics by age 14, or who have no menstrual period by the age of 16 regardless of whether secondary sexual characteristics are present or not.

1. If a patient has the *absence of breast tissue*, but *has a uterus*, then the presumption can be made that there is no estrogen being produced because of hypothalamic-pituitary failure or lack of ovarian follicles, but the patient should have a normal female karyotype with a normal mullerian system. In this case you would test for FSH and LH. If the **FSH** is *low*, then consider hypothalamic-pituitary failure, and if it is *elevated* then consider a lack of ovarian follicles. If the **LH** is *low*, then it is probably due to hypogonadotropic hypogonadism, and if it is *normal* or *elevated* then consider gonadal dysgenesis.
2. When an individual has evidence of breast tissue, but an *absent uterus*, the presumption can be made that there is endogenous estrogen production, presence of responsive ovarian follicles, and a functional hypothalamic-pituitary-ovarian axis. The absence of the uterus suggests that the patient is chromosomally a *male* with testicular feminization or androgen insensitivity, or chromosomally female but the mullerian system failed to develop. To distinguish between the two, you must test the level of testosterone. If there are normal male levels, then it is the former case, and if there are normal female levels, then it is the latter one. These can also be distinguished by karyotyping the individual.
3. When there is an absence of *both* breast tissue and the uterus, then the presumption is that there is failure of the hypothalamic-pituitary axis or lack of ovarian follicles and the individual is a karyotypic male with testicular feminization or androgen insensitivity, or a karyotypic female with failed development of the mullerian system. This example is a very rare occurrence, and karyotyping, along with FSH and testosterone levels, is needed to identify the problem. These cases are present in agonadism, 17,20-desmolase deficiency, and 17-hydroxylase deficiency.
4. If the individual *has* breast tissue *and* a uterus, then it can be presumed that there was endogenous estrogen production, presence of responsive ovarian follicles, a functional hypothalamic-pituitary-ovarian axis, and

a female karyotype with a developed mullerian system. The current problem involves either reproductive tract outflow anomalies (such as vaginal agenesis, transverse vaginal septum, and imperforate hymen) or it is a hypothalamic-pituitary-ovarian axis problem.

To evaluate what the problem is, a *progesterone challenge test* can be done. A positive test will show *withdrawal bleeding* and an estrogen level *greater* than 40 pg/ml, and it can be assumed that the ovarian follicles are functional.

Then, the *LH level* is checked, and if it is moderately elevated consider polycystic ovarian syndrome. If it is low, consider hypothalamic dysfunction. (A negative test will have no withdrawal bleeding and inadequate levels of estrogen.)

If the *FSH* is low, then consider hypothalamic-pituitary failure. If the FSH is *very high*, consider ovarian failure.

### Secondary amenorrhea

This refers to a female who has been menstruating, but has the absence of menstruation for 6 months, or more. With amenorrhea, *always* consider pregnancy.

In secondary amenorrhea, if the individual had a female karyotype, functional mullerian system, ovarian follicles, and functional hypothalamic-pituitary axis at the time of normal menses, then either there have been *mullerian system changes* (such as pregnancy or uterine adhesions), ovarian failure, or hypothalamic-pituitary-ovarian axis dysfunction (such as elevated prolactin with galactorrhea, medications, stress, exercise, or polycystic ovarian syndrome).

As you may recall, drugs such as tranquilizers are *dopamine antagonists* that block dopamine inhibition of prolactin and deplete hypothalamic catecholamines. Tricyclic antidepressants act by blocking catecholamine re-uptake, reserpine depletes catecholamine stores, and methyldopa blocks tyrosine conversion to dopamine. To evaluate, a proper clinical assessment is necessary. Test the patient's levels of prolactin, TSH, LH, and FSH to properly diagnose. The *progesterone challenge* may be employed using the same rationale as in primary amenorrhea. If the test is negative for a bleed, then you must consider premature ovarian failure with elevated FSH and treat the patient as if she were postmenopausal or experiencing hypothalamic-pituitary failure with normal or decreased FSH. Imaging of the *sella turcica* should be done to rule out *craniopharyngioma*. If the test is positive for a bleed, then you would use OCPs, dexamethasone, and spironolactone (if the androgens are elevated) to induce bleeding monthly. In the case of polycystic ovaries, there will be an *increased* LH. If the LH is *normal* then consider hypothalamic dysfunction, and its cause needs to be ruled out.

### DYSMENORRHEA

This is the presence of *painful* menstrual cramps and is classified as primary or secondary.

### Primary dysmenorrhea

*Primary* dysmenorrhea refers to painful menstrual cramps with **no** underlying visible pelvic pathology to account for the pain. Onset occurs within two years of menarche and just prior to or at menses, lasting 48 to 72 h. It may be associated with nausea and vomiting, fatigue, diarrhea, and headache. Etiology can be related to excessive myometrial contractions, decreased uterine blood flow, uterine ischemia, and excessive endometrial prostaglandin production of $PGF_{2a}$ and $PG_{E2}$.

Management includes reassurance, nonsteroidal anti-inflammatory agents, OCPs, psychotherapy, and avoidance of surgical procedures such as D & C, presacral neurectomy, and uterosacral ligament transection.

### Secondary dysmenorrhea

*Secondary* dysmenorrhea is painful menstrual cramps *with* a readily identifiable pelvic lesion responsible for the pain. The onset is usually at about 20 to 30 years of age and may be associated with dyspareunia, infertility, and abnormal bleeding. Etiology can be related to endometriosis, pelvic inflammation, adenomyosis, leiomyomata, pelvic congestion syndrome, and ovarian cysts. Its treatment is usually directed toward the primary problem.

## ABNORMAL UTERINE BLEEDING

Abnormal uterine bleeding is a phrase that describes *pathologic alterations* in the normal pattern of *menstrual flow*.

**Dysfunctional uterine bleeding** is the most common type of abnormal genital tract bleeding in adolescents and adults. Abnormalities take several forms, including excessive flow, prolonged flow, and intermenstrual bleeding. Dysfunctional uterine bleeding (DUB) is reserved for *anorulatory* bleeding (absence of any organic disease). DUB is considered a "diagnosis of exclusion."

**Organic causes** can be further broken down into **systemic causes** (such as coagulopathies, hepatic disease, renal disease, obesity, steroid hormones, anticoagulants, chemotherapeutic drugs, and endocrine diseases), and **local diseases** (such as leiomyomas, uterine or cervical polyps and endometrial hyperplasia, PID, IUDs, hormone producing ovarian tumors, and pregnancy).

**Nonorganic abnormal uterine bleeding** encompasses endocrine disorders and aberrant reproductive hormone secretion. The persistent failure to ovulate, which results in dysfunctional uterine bleeding, is responsible for the majority of cases of abnormal bleeding. The predominant cause of anovulation is altered neuroendocrinologic function. Abnormal uterine bleeding can also be described by how much bleeding occurs.

**Menorrhagia,** or **hypermenorrhea,** is bleeding that is cyclic and regular but excessive in amount and/or duration and may be due to pregnancy, submucous myomas, or hyperplasia/carcinoma.

**Hypomenorrhea** is unusually light or diminished flow and is caused by OCP usage, narrowed hymen or cervical canal, and Asherman's syndrome.

**Polymenorrhea** occurs with increased bleeding (less than 21-day cycles) and is often associated with anovulation and seldom results from shortened luteal phase (except in perimenopause).

**Oligomenorrhea** occurs with decreased bleeding (greater than 35-day cycles) and is associated with anovulation.

**Metrorrhagia** is intermenstrual bleeding at any time between menses and is normally associated with ovulatory mid-cycle bleeding. This may be caused by cervical or endometrial polyps, or cervical or endometrial carcinoma, or may be normal in 10 percent of women.

**Menometrorrhagia** is irregular menstruation in frequency and in excessive amount and may be frequently associated with organic pathology, particularly if sudden onset.

To evaluate someone with abnormal uterine bleeding history and examination, think about: "Is the patient pregnant?" or "Is there a mass or tenderness on exam?" *Cytology* may be excellent for diagnosing a cervical lesion but is unreliable for assessing the pathology of the uterus, oviducts, or ovaries. An *endometrial biopsy* could be helpful for diagnosing hormonal status. A *hysterosalpingogram* can potentially outline an intrauterine lesion such as endometrial polyp, but has the potential for spreading malignant cells. *Hysteroscopy* can be helpful by direct visualization of lesions and the potential for taking a *biopsy* is available. A *pelvic ultrasound* may be helpful in the identification of a pelvic mass. An ultrasound can be combined with *hysterosonography* to visualize uterine lesions.

#### ENDOMETRIOSIS
Endometriosis refers to endometrial tissue in an ectopic location exclusive of the myometrium with ectopic endometrial glands and stroma as well as evidence of menstrual cyclicity. It is almost exclusively confined to women in their reproductive years and the diagnosis is typically made in the age range of 25 to 40. The mean onset is at age 20 but symptoms can also be experienced in the teenage years.

Endometriosis has been postulated to result from either retrograde menstruation where endometrial tissue implants in ectopic locations, or from substances released from shed endometrium inducing undifferentiated mesenchyme to form endometriosis. Other postulates include genetic predisposition, immunologic dysfunction, and activation of embryonic cell rests.

Symptoms may include: infertility, dysmenorrhea (most commonly reported), dyspareunia, noncyclic lower abdominal pain and backaches, dyschezia, dysuria, and urinary urgency. However, some patients may be asymptomatic.

*Laparoscopy* is the method of choice for diagnosing endometriosis, and can also be used in the treatment as well. Management also includes expectant treatment for mild to moderate disease, surgical therapy including: conservative methods like lysis of adhesions, suspension of uterus and ovaries, partial omentectomy by laparotomy or laparoscopy, sharp dissection, cautery, or electrocoagulation of endometriotic implants, presacral neurectomy, and uterosacral transection. More definitive methods include hysterectomy and, in some instances, bilateral salpingo-oophorectomy.

Pharmacologic therapy includes: danazol, progesterone agents, gestrinone (an antiprogestational steroid), OCPs used either in a 21 days on and 7 days off fashion or in a continuous fashion, and gonadotropin-releasing hormone analogs, such as naferelin and leuprolide to down-regulate the pituitary gland. *Combination* medical-surgical treatment can be carried out with pharmacologic therapy administered either before or after the operation, with the main improvement of symptoms coming from pain.

### ADENOMYOSIS

This is the presence of normal-appearing endometrial glands and stroma within the myometrium of the uterus. It is almost always accompanied by *muscular hypertrophy* within the uterine wall, and frequently is associated with *fibroid tumors* of the uterus or *endometriosis.*

The most common symptoms are: pelvic pain, dysmenorrhea, and abnormally increased menstrual flow. It is generally thought to be estrogen responsive and thus symptoms may decrease after menopause. The age at diagnosis is usually in the later reproductive years, 30 to 40 years old, and it is shown to increase with increasing age from 20 to 50 year olds. Diagnosis requires biopsy or hysterectomy. Medical treatment with hormonal therapy has only shown to be effective in 20 percent of patients using progesterone therapy. Surgical treatment by hysterectomy is the only definitive treatment.

### PREMENSTRUAL SYNDROME (PMS) OR LATE-LUTEAL PHASE SYNDROME

This is a clinical syndrome wherein women experience the cyclic appearance of emotional and/or physical symptoms that worsen as menstruation approaches and rapidly dissipate with menstrual flow. Symptoms are experienced in the second half of the cycle and should be present over at least three consecutive cycles for diagnosis. Symptoms include: fluid retention, breast tenderness, headache, abdominal distention, nausea, vomiting, and mood changes. The cause is unknown, but several hypotheses such as neurotransmitter dysfunction, steroid hormone imbalance, prostaglandin imbalance, fluid retention, vitamin deficiency, mineral deficiency, and psychosomatic illness have been cited (but not accepted).

The diagnosis is really a clinical one. Management includes: reassurance, diet modification such as decreased caffeine and alcohol intake at appropriate times, exercise, which when done regularly improves dysmenorrhea and reduces symptoms, and stress reduction.

For complaints of dysmenorrhea and menorrhagia, birth control pills, nonsteroidal anti-inflammatory drugs, and gonadotropin releasing hormone agonists can be used. As a last resort (if fertility is not of concern), a hysterectomy can be done. Furthermore, spironolactone, decreasing the use of tobacco (since it stimulates ADH), and *evening primrose oil* can be used for problems with fluid retention. Evening primrose oil may also be used for depression and mastalgia. Danazol is also useful for mastalgia as well as for emotional symptoms. For treatment of emotional symptoms (like depression and anxiety) consider: GnRH agonists—such as leuprolide or nafarelin—in conjunction with premarin; alprazolam, naltrexone, and serotonin-enhancing drugs—such as fluoxetine and buspirone.

# Sexually Transmitted Diseases and the Abnormal Pap

# 7

## SEXUALLY TRANSMITTED DISEASES

STDs are used to denote those infections that usually are transmitted by intimate contact between two people. The most common infections transmitted by sexual contact include: chlamydia, gonorrhea, herpes, HIV, and syphilis. Although hepatitis B virus is often transmitted via sexual contact it will not be discussed because it does not have any gynecologic manifestations. Most common modes of transmission include intimate contact, mother to offspring transmission, fomites such as moist towels or "sex toys," and contaminated blood products. It is important to remember that for all STDs, the partner(s) should also be treated.

### CHLAMYDIA

Chlamydia infection is caused by the organism *Chlamydia trachomatis*, and is the most commonly sexually transmitted genital infection in women. Risk factors include: being sexually active and younger than 20 years old, having multiple sexual partners, having a new sexual partner within 3 months, non-use of barrier contraceptives, lower socioeconomic status, and history of other STDs.

Frequently, women are asymptomatic even when salpingitis is present. The cervix is usually friable and inflamed. Cell culture is the gold standard for diagnosis with 100 percent specificity but we may soon find DNA probe analysis common because it takes less time to diagnose, approximately 1 h, and the sensitivity is >90 percent and specificity is >95 percent. Complications include: salpingitis leading to infertility due to tubal obstruction, ectopic pregnancy, pelvic pain, dyspareunia, neonatal infection leading to inclusion conjunctivitis and otitis media, and obstetrical problems such as premature delivery and postpartum endometritis. Currently the infection is most commonly treated with *azythromicin,* 1gm taken orally at one time. One may also use *doxycycline* or *tetracycline* for 7 days to treat.

## GONORRHEA

This is caused by *Neisseria gonorrheae*, a gram-*negative diplococcus* bacteria. Typically, this organism can be recovered from the urethra, cervix, anal canal, and the pharynx. Seventy-five percent of women will be infected after exposure to an infected sexual partner and 30 percent will also have concomitant *chlamydia infections.*

Early on the women may be asymptomatic if the infection is pharyngeal, cervical, or anorectal, but there may be some purulent cervical discharge, urinary frequency, dysuria, and rectal discomfort. The vaginal, vulvar, and perineal areas may have inflammation, discharge, itching and burning. Late clinical findings may include bartholin gland abscess; disseminated infection such as polyarthralgia, tenosynovitis, dermatitis, purulent arthritis, pericarditis, endocarditis, and meningitis; ophthalmic infection such as conjunctivitis and ophthalmia neonatorum; and vulvovaginitis in children. Diagnosis is by culture on *Thayer-Martin media.* Treatment is with *cefoxitin* 2 g IM or *ceftriaxone* 250 mg IM.

## HERPES SIMPLEX VIRUS

Herpes Simplex Virus infection, or HSV, is a DNA virus that is acquired by mucocutaneous contact and establishes permanent, incurable latency in the sensory ganglia. In a primary outbreak the symptoms appear 3 to 7 days after exposure and may have some prodromal symptoms such as paresthesias and *burning.*

Physical findings may include: fever; malaise; adenopathy; vesicles that are clear, tender, and painful on the vulva and perianal skin; and asymptomatic vesicles on the vaginal mucosa and ectocervix. Thirty percent of the cases of primary HSV progress to a *recurrent syndrome* where the virus migrates up the nerve fiber to the dorsal root ganglia and remains dormant until activated again, then travels back down the nerve fiber to the previously infected site. Viral culture is the definitive way to diagnose. There is **no** effective cure for this infection but topical or oral *acyclovir,* a purine analog, may shorten the frequency and severity. The patient should abstain from sexual contact while lesions are active and present.

## HUMAN IMMUNODEFICIENCY VIRUS

HIV infection is a *single*-stranded **R**NA-enveloped **retro**virus that uses *reverse transcriptase* to make a DNA copy of itself, and then integrates into the host's genome. The mode of transmission is *sexual contact* with an infected partner, *exposure* to infected blood or blood products, and exposure to used IV drug needles with infected virus. An infected mother may transmit the virus to the fetus.

*High risk groups* include: IV drug users who use dirty or shared needles, individuals with multiple sexual partners, bisexual individuals, those with a history of other STDs, those who travel to or from endemic areas, those engaging in sexual practices not using barrier protective methods, and those individuals who received blood transfusions prior to 1985.

To be diagnosed with AIDS, an HIV infected person must develop an opportunistic infection, Kaposi's sarcoma, dementia encephalopathy, wasting syndrome, a CD4 count **<200**/mm$^3$, or invasive cervical carcinoma.

There is **no** current cure for this disease and the focus is on *prevention* with such measures as abstinence, mutually monogamous sex between HIV-negative partners, "safer" sex practices (such as use of latex condoms with *nonoxynol-9* and reduced number of sexual partners, avoidance of previously used needles, and taking *universal precautions* when dealing with any body fluids).

HIV testing is usually for HIV-1 antibodies using the **ELISA**, an enzyme-linked immunosorbent assay, as a *screening* test for the antibodies. If the ELISA is positive, then a **Western blot assay** is done to *confirm* if the test is positive or reactive.

*Treatment* is directed at suppression of viral replication in patients with **CD4** counts **<500**/ml by using **AZT** (zidovudine), **DDI** (didanosine), **DDC** (zalcitabine), and prophylaxis for opportunistic infections with **SMZ-TMP** (sulfamethoxazole/trimethoprim) and nebulized **pentamidine** for *Pneumocystis carinii*, and **diflucan** for antifungal protection. **Rifabutin** has recently been approved for *Mycobacterium avium intracellulare* prophylaxis.

### SYPHILIS

Syphilis infection is by the spirochete *Treponema pallidum*. Primary syphilis manifests as a vulvar or vaginal chancre 10 to 60 days after exposure that heals in 3 to 9 weeks, and also as painless lymph nodes on exam. The latent period appears in 8 weeks, 3 to 6 weeks after the chancre. *Secondary* syphillis has systemic manifestations of generalized adenopathy and condylomata lata which are highly contagious perineal exophytic excrescences that ulcerate. This stage passes spontaneously 2 to 6 weeks into latency. Tertiary syphillis has diffuse organ system involvement and gummas that are necrotic, ulcerative nodules.

Screening is done through serology using the RPR or the VDRL test, which have 15 percent false positive rates. The FTA-ABS test is used to confirm the diagnosis because it is a treponema-specific test. Treatment is usually with **penicillin** given intramuscularly and if the disease is latent and present for over 1 year, then the doses are repeated for three weeks.

---

## THE PAPANICOLAOU (PAP) SMEAR

The Pap smear is a *screening* test for *cervical disease* and abnormal cell pathology. Pap smears are the most prevalent method of the detection of CIN, cervical intraepithelial neoplasia, which displays no symptoms or physical signs, and is undetectable by routine physical exam. Usually, screening for cervical cytology is done *annually* on all women who are or have been sexually active. Women with cytologic abnormalities are generally evaluated using colposcopy and colposcopically directed biopsies.

*Colposcopy* involves the careful inspection of the cervix using a stereoscopic binocular microscope called a colposcope. These are used to distinguish columnar epithelium, native squamous epithelium, and metaplastic squamous epithelium.

Usually, an *endocervical curettage* (ECC) is performed after the colposcopy unless the patient is pregnant. Abnormal changes of cervical topography probably require presence of a carcinogen such as cigarette smoke, factors transmitted through intercourse at a young age due to an immature transformation zone, and human papillomavirus, or **HPV,** types **6, 11, 16**, and **18,** which is thought to be associated with—if not transmitted by—*sexual contact.*

Risk factors for cervical dysplasia and carcinoma include: early age of sexual intercourse, multiple sexual partners, early age of marriage, *early* age of pregnancy, high parity, low socioeconomic status, divorce, and *cigarette smoking.* The comparison of the different classification systems for cervical cytology is listed in Table 7-1.

Management of the abnormal pap depends on the cytologic classification obtained and the choice of the clinician. Different types of therapy are listed below with their failure rates:

### CRYOTHERAPY

This is a painless out-patient procedure done in the office with nitrous oxide that is inexpensive and leaves no scarring, and has a 10 to 20 percent failure rate. Its disadvantages include: not being able to selectively target only dysplastic areas, destruction of the transformation zone or T-zone due to the subcutaneous junction moving into the endocervical canal, and no histologic specimen.

**Table 7-1**   Cancer Classification Systems

| Class System | CIN System | Bethesda System |
|---|---|---|
| Class I: Normal | Normal | Within normal limits |
| Class II: Inflammation | Inflammatory | Inflammatory: with/without atypia |
| Class III: Mild/ moderate dysplasia | CIN I or II | Low-grade SIL |
| Class IV: Severe dysplasia/CIS | CIN III | High-grade SIL |
| Class V: Suggestive of cancer | Suggestive of cancer | Squamous cell cancer |

NOTE: CIS, carcinoma in situ; CIN, cervical intraepithelial neoplasia; SIL, squamous intraepithelial lesion

## CO$_2$ LASER

This laser therapy has a 5 to 10 percent failure rate, and can give precise destruction of only the dysplastic areas with minimal scarring and no damage to the T-zone. It can be used to ablate the T-zone or as a tool for cone biopsies. This procedure can be expensive because it requires operating room time and general anesthesia. It can be *painful*, and there is still no histologic specimen obtained.

### ELECTROCAUTERY

This has a low failure rate of about 5 percent, but it is also expensive (requiring OR time and general anesthesia), and has no histologic specimen—and may even *cause* cervical stenosis.

### LOOP ELECTRODIATHERMY EXCISION PROCEDURE (LEEP)

LEEP uses a small, fine, wire loop attached to an electrosurgical generator and provides a histologic specimen and is relatively *painless*. It can be done as an out-patient procedure in the clinician's office. However, due to the electrocautery effect, the margins from the specimen obtained may be obliterated, and it therefore may be difficult to distinguish if they are clear or not.

### CERVICAL CONE BIOPSY

Cone biopsy has a very *high* cure rate and *provides* a histologic specimen. This procedure should be performed in the OR due to the risk of *bleeding* and *infection* (a lot of tissue is taken). There is also a risk of *cervical incompetence* and *cervical stenosis* after having the procedure done.

The indications for cone biopsy include: T-zone not fully visualized by colposcopy, positive ECC, significant discrepancy between the pap and the colpo biopsy, biopsy reveals microinvasive squamous cell carcinoma, or biopsy reveals adenocarcinoma in situ.

The **FIGO** (International Federation of Gynecologists and Obstetricians) clinical staging for cervical carcinoma is as follows:

**Stage 0**    Carcinoma *in situ* confined to the epithelium only

**Stage I**    Invasion strictly confined to the cervix
*IA1*    Minimal microscopically evident stromal invasion
*IA2*    Microscopic invasion ≤ 5mm, with horizontal spread ≤ 7mm
*IB*    All others

**Stage II**    Invasion beyond cervix but not to the pelvic wall or lower ⅓ of the vagina
*IIA*    Parametria not involved
*IIB*    Parametria involved

**Stage III**    Invasion to the pelvic wall or lower ⅓ of the vagina
*IIIA*    Pelvic wall not involved, but involvement of the lower ⅓ of the vagina
*IIIB*    Pelvic wall involvement, or hydronephrosis or nonfunctioning kidney due to tumor

**Stage IV** Invasion beyond the true pelvis or mucosa of the bladder or rectum
*IVA*      Spread to the adjacent organs
*IVB*      Spread to distant organs

Early *symptoms* of **cervical carcinoma** may include: vaginal bleeding, postcoital bleeding, and acyclic irregular bleeding. However, the patient may be asymptomatic with discovery by routine physical exam or cytologic screening. Symptoms of *advanced disease* may include: malodorous vaginal discharge, weight loss, flank pain, unilateral pain or edema of the lower extremities, dysuria or hematuria, rectal bleeding or constipation, and profuse hemorrhage, uremia, and profound inanination.

Management may include: *surgery* such as a *radical hysterectomy* with *bilateral pelvic lymphadenectomy* (for patients whose disease is confined to the cervix and closely adjacent tissues); *irradiation, which* is most effective against regional disease; and *chemotherapy,* which with cytotoxic agents may be used to control distant disease. Also, chemotherapy may be simultaneously with *radiation therapy* to potentiate the radiation effect, or in a neoadjuvant manner, to shrink the tumor prior to surgery or radiation therapy.

The most common type of *cervical carcinoma* is **squamous cell** *carcinoma,* which is what the above classification for staging is based upon. Other cervical neoplasms include: *adenocarcinoma* with an incidence from 5 to 20 percent; *adenosquamous* carcinoma, which is prone to early hematogenous metastasis; *small cell cancer,* which originates from the APUD (amine precursor uptake and decarboxylation) cell system; *verrucous carcinoma,* which is treatable by total or modified radical hysterectomy; and *cervical sarcoma,* which is treatable surgically when confined to the cervix but does have a preponderance for hematogenous spread. Metastatic disease to the cervix has been reported for ovary, fallopian tube, colon, and breast, but the cervix is considered to be an infrequent site for metastases.

# Benign Lesions of the Genital Tract 8

**Vulvar benign disease** can be divided into those with infectious, atrophic, dystrophic, allergic, and trauma-related causes.

## INFECTIOUS CAUSES

These include *viral, bacterial, fungal,* and *pubic lice.*

### VIRAL INFECTIONS

These include genital warts or condylomas, which are characterized by one or more noticeable, but painless growths with variable size, but may be pruritic and painful. *Genital herpes* is usually caused by HSV type **2.** *Molluscum contagiosum* is an uncommon disease caused by a poxvirus and is usually spread by sexual contact.

Genital warts can be treated using *TCA* (trichloracetic acid), which chemically cauterizes the tissue, podophyllotoxin, which acts by poisoning the mitotic spindle, and cryotherapy or electrocautery, which causes local destruction of the tissue. *Laser surgery* is highly effective for extensive, persistent, or recurrent condylomas and is the treatment of choice, and *interferon* may be injected directly into persistent or recurrent lesions to act immunologically. *Acyclovir* is used for HSV, but does not cure the disease. Treatment for molluscum contagiosum is removal through *curettage* followed by application of *Monsel's solution* or by topical application of phenol or TCA.

### BACTERIAL INFECTIONS

These include *Staphylococcus folliculitis,* which is treated with antibiotics and local heat; *cellulitis,* which may be from gram-positive cocci or may be polymicrobial and treated with antibiotics; *necrotizing fasciitis,* which requires wide debridement and antibiotic therapy; and *hidradenitis suppurativa,* which is a mixed infection involving the apocine glands of the vulva and is characterized by multiple pustules and abscesses and is treated with broad-spectrum antibiotics combined with extensive surgical debridement.

*Bartholin's abscess* is a common vulvar manifestation of the lower genital tract (caused by *Gonorrhea*) that is treated primarily by incision and drainage or by marsupialization or excision of the bartholin's gland for recurrent disease.

*Chancroid* is an infection by sexual transmission of *Haemophilus ducreyi* that causes labial and perineal ulcers often with inguinal adenopathy with abscess formation and suppuration. It is treated with erythromycin four times a day for ten days or with a single dose of ceftriaxone given intramuscularly. Lymphogranuloma venereum is a sexually transmitted disease caused by the L-serrovariant of *Chlamydia trichomatis* and is more commonly found in tropical areas. Doxycycline given twice a day for two weeks is the usual treatment and incision and drainage should be avoided because it can lead to chronically draining sinuses.

*Granuloma inguinale* is caused by *Calymmatobacterium granulomatis,* and starts out as an ulcerated papule with progressive spread and surrounding cellulitis that is treated with tetracycline or erythromycin for three weeks.

### FUNGAL INFECTIONS
These are usually due to *Candida albicans* and can be treated with an antifungal medication such as terazol cream or ointment or diflucan orally.

### PUBIC LICE
**Pubic lice** are often transmitted sexually; the patient may experience pruritus, excoriation, and erythema. Upon careful inspection of the mons with a magnifying glass, *small white eggs,* called "nits," of the lice can be seen. *Permethrin cream* (Nix) or *benzene hydrochloride lotion* (Kwell) can be used topically twice at 10 day intervals for cure. Potentially contaminated clothing and bedding should be *washed* in hot water or dry cleaned to *prevent re-infection* and treatment of *all sexual partners* is mandatory.

---

## ATROPHY OF THE VULVA

Vulvar atrophy occurs in most women *at menopause* due to the withdrawal of estrogen and is associated with thinning epithelium, loss of subcutaneous fat, and atrophy of the perineal muscles. If patients are asymptomatic then no therapy is required. For symptoms of pruritis and dyspareunia, estrogen either topically or systemically has been shown to be effective.

---

## VULVAR DYSTROPHIES

These are *benign* dermatologic conditions with *pruritus* as a common symptom. There are two types of dystrophy currently recognized, which are defined on the basis of their histologic appearance. All lesions should be biopsied to guide treatment and exclude neoplasia.

### SQUAMOUS CELL HYPERPLASIA OR HYPERTROPHIC DYSTROPHY
This is a chronic dermatitis that may be related to chronic irritation. *White patches* may be seen on the vulva, often accompanied by *lichenification* and

excoriation. Treatment includes: keeping the skin clean and dry, avoiding all chemical irritants, and *triamcinolone acetate* steroid cream at 0.1% is used initially two to three times a day until signs and symptoms resolve. Then, *prophylaxis* with hydrocortisone 1% cream is used when symptoms are controlled.

### LICHEN SCLEROSUS

This has an unknown etiology, but usually occurs in postmenopausal women, although women of any age can be affected. Patients usually experience *pruritus or burning* and usually present with hypopigmented *white lesions* on the vulva, with thinning of the skin and atrophy of the labia minora.

Testosterone proprionate 2% ointment in petrolatum jelly is applied topically two to three times daily, and has been somewhat effective in treating lichen sclerosus, but some patients require biweekly treatments for years to avoid recurrence. Hydrocortisone cream 1% is sometimes applied two to three times a day initially until pruritus resolves. Surgery should be reserved for lysis of labial adhesions and introital stenosis.

## ALLERGIC VULVITIS

Allergic vulvitis, such as a *contact dermatitis*, can occur in response to a variety of allergens and semen and may mimic vulvar infections. Many soaps, perfumes, dyes, douches, and feminine hygiene products contain irritants that can initiate vulvitis. Pruritus, pain, and exudate are common symptoms. Elimination of the allergen and topical steroid usage is the usual therapy.

## VULVAR TRAUMA

Trauma can occur during falls, childbirth, rape, or coitus. The cardinal symptom is local pain. Treatment includes meticulous control of bleeding, and if there is an enlarging hematoma, it should be explored and packed.

## BENIGN VAGINAL AND CERVICAL DISORDERS

These usually are caused by viral, fungal, protozoan, or bacterial infections. Vaginal discharge and pruritus are symptoms shared by all causes of vaginitis-cervicitis.

**HSV and HPV** are the two known viruses that infect the vagina and cervix. The diagnosis and treatment is similar to that in other areas of the genital tract.

**Candida albicans** is the major fungal pathogen and has pruritus as the major symptom. Diagnosis is by the KOH prep and wet prep, and treatment is with any of the antifungal creams or oral preparations.

**Trichomonas vaginalis** usually has a frothy discharge with a foul odor. The wet prep will show motile flagellated organisms and treatment is with metronidazole.

**Gonorrhea** may have a cervical discharge and can only be diagnosed by culture. Ceftriaxone is the treatment of choice.

**Chlamydia** may have a mucopurulent discharge and cervical erosion and rapid DNA probe testing is frequently used to diagnose. Azithromycin, doxycycline, or erythromycin can be used to treat it.

**Bacterial vaginosis** has a thin gray discharge with a fishy odor and is diagnosed by wet prep. Metronidazole gel used at night for 7 days is the usual treatment of choice.

### Toxic shock syndrome

This syndrome is caused by *Staphylococci* production of *toxins* or epidermal exfoliative toxins. It is related to the use of *vaginal tampons* that have not been changed frequently enough. The symptoms include: sudden high *fever*, flu-like symptoms (sore throat, headache, diarrhea), hypotension, and a "sunburn" rash or *exfoliation* of the palmar sides of hands and feet. It is important to have prophylactic frequent changing of tampons. Treatment includes: remove the intravaginal tampon, drain any abscess, supportive care (for hypotension), and parenteral antibiotics for penicillinase-resistant Staphylococcus aureus (like IV Oxacillin).

---

## INTRAEPITHELIAL NEOPLASMS OF THE LOWER GENITAL TRACT

There are three types, depending on the organ that harbors the premalignant condition. Cellular changes begin just superficial to the basement membrane and involve more of the thickness of the epithelium as the condition progresses. The grade is based on the severity of the nuclear abnormalities and the amount of mitotic activity, as well as the proportion of the epithelium involved.

Cervical intraepithelial neoplasia (**CIN**) has four grades:

> CIN I—or mild dysplasia, involves the innermost one-third of the cervical epithelium
> CIN II—or moderate dysplasia, involves the innermost two-thirds of the epithelium
> CIN III—or severe dysplasia, involves more than two-thirds of the thickness of the epithelium but not the full thickness
> CIS—or carcinoma in situ, involves the full thickness

Vaginal intraepithelial neoplasia (**VaIN**), and vulvar intraepithelial neoplasia (**VIN**), are graded and treated in a similar way (refer to section on the *abnormal pap*). VaIN II or III is treated with surgical excision, laser surgery, or radiation. VIN I is managed like vulvar condyloma, whereas VIN II or III is treated by laser surgery, wide local excision, skinning vulvectomy with split-thickness skin graft, or a simple vulvectomy. The more advanced diseases of intraepithelial neoplasms are treated more vigorously because of their potential for becoming cancerous lesions.

## ENDOMETRIAL POLYPS

These polyps may take the form of sessile or pedunculated lesions. They are composed of normal endometrial glands, which are dilated, and stroma that may have a cellular, hyperplastic appearance (similar to that of the endometrial hyperplasias). They can cause metrorrhagia, increased perimenopausal bleeding, postmenopausal bleeding, and, rarely, prolapse through the cervix. Hysteroscopy and D & C can both be used in the diagnosis and treatment of polyps. If the polyps are malignant, then they should be treated following the guidelines for any uterine cancer of the same histologic type.

## ENDOMETRIAL HYPERPLASIA

This covers a histologically-defined spectrum of changes in the endometrium, ranging from benign to precancerous. *Cystic hyperplasia* is characterized by tall columnar or cuboidal cells, and rarely progresses to carcinoma. *Adenomatous hyperplasia* has complex glands containing branches and buds, and are lined with columnar cells that show no nuclear atypia and can occasionally progress to carcinoma. *Atypical adenomatous hyperplasia* consists of complex glands separated by discernible stroma and as many as half of these lesions progress to carcinoma if left untreated. Back to back glands with no intervening stroma and glandular lesions with a cribiform pattern are suggestive of carcinoma.

*Endometrial hyperplasia* usually presents either as postmenopausal bleeding or as an increase in *bleeding*. Diagnosis is by endometrial biopsy, D & C, or hysteroscopy. If the patient is **pre**menopausal and wishes to conceive, but is anovulatory, then ovulation is induced (or, if she does not wish to conceive, she is placed on a progesterone rich OCP), and D & C or hysteroscopy is repeated in 6 months regardless. If the patient is **post**menopausal, then a hysterectomy is performed on those women with atypical hyperplasia or if she has cystic or adenomatous hyperplasia, hormone therapy or danozol may be used. If hormonal therapy fails, then D & C or hysteroscopy-directed biopsy are done after 6 months.

## UTERINE LEIOMYOMAS (FIBROIDS)

Uterine leiomyomas (fibroids) (Fig. 8-1) are smooth muscle tumors, occurring in about 30 percent of all females, usually <40 years old. These fibroids are the most common lesions of the uterine wall. They are solid, round, benign, whorled tumors that are thought to arise from a single cell. Fibroids

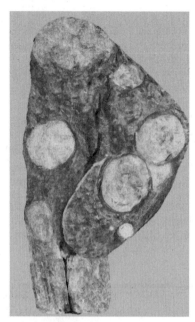

**Figure 8-1**   Fibroids or leiomyomas of the uterus. Leiomyomas are round, rubbery nodules of benign masses of smooth muscle cells. They are the most common tumors in women. Usually present in women over 30, and may be asymptomatic or with irregular, painful bleeding.

are usually found *encapsulated* within a periphery of normal uterine smooth muscle. Fibroids may be found submucousally, intramurally, subserousally, or intraligamentously in the uterine cavity. They may also be found in the cervix and peritoneum. Fibroids are the most common reason for surgery. They grow large and are considered benign, but have minimal malignant potential. There is an increase in African-American and estrogen-dependent (OCPs) women.

Fibroids also appear as polypoid lesions within the endometrial cavity. Symptoms may include severe *dysmenorrhea* and *menometrorrhagia* with the bleeding caused by superficial ulceration of the fibroids (or by compromise of the ability of the highly vascularized area surrounding the base of the lesion to contract during menses).

Fibroids present as: asymptomatic pelvic pressure, congestion, bloating, heaviness, and frequent urination. Uterine fibroids are characterized by *abdominal swelling, increased* menstrual bleeding, and *pain* during intercourse. Usually there is NO pain unless a pregnancy occurs. Complications include: infertility, pregnancy complications, and malignant degeneration.

Diagnosis can be done by physical exam and ultrasound, hysteroscopy and D & C (which are both also used to treat them), and hysterectomy can be an excellent alternative in older women who have no plans for childbearing (perform a *fractional D & C* to rule out *endometrial carcinoma*).

The treatment is *observation*. Then, myomectomy or surgery if there is continued bleeding. Medical management includes: GnRH agonists as an adjunct to surgery, relieve pain, decrease the size of myomas and decrease the bleeding, correct the anemia, and decrease the intraoperative blood loss. These patients may not respond with amenorrhea when treated with *gonadotropin releasing hormone agonists*.

Most fibroids do NOT require treatment, but surgical removal of the fibroids include: (1) *hysterectomy* (remove the uterus), (2) *myomectomy* (remove fibroids), and (3) a new possibility still being reviewed includes *uterine artery embolization*. This embolization technique allows a catheter to enter the artery, and inject plastics to clog the artery. This stops the blood flow *to the fibroid*, but the uterus maintains adequate circulation.

## POLYCYSTIC OVARY SYNDROME (PCOS) AND ANOVULATION

These are the most common forms of ovulatory failure. Elevation of serum androgens, unbalanced serum LH elevation, and ultrasound evidence of ovarian enlargement with multiple midsize follicles are reliable diagnostic findings. Eighty percent of women with PCOS will respond to clomiphene citrate by ovulating.

## PELVIC INFLAMMATORY DISEASE (PID) AND TUBO-OVARIAN ABSCESS

These may present with *insidious* (few or no symptoms) or *acute onset* of bilateral lower abdominal and pelvic pain, a sensation of pelvic pressure with back pain radiating down the legs, and nausea and/or vomiting, with cervical motion tenderness ("chandelier sign"), adnexal tenderness, purulent discharge, and abdominal tenderness on exam. Infection is due to ascending infection from the lower tract and results in purulent salpingitis with pus into the peritoneal cavity.

Classic invaders include: gonorrhea, chlamydia, mycoplasma, and ureaplasma. Criteria for in-patient treatment includes abscess, temperature >39°C, septicemia, failed out-patient management, and first episode in a nulligravid patient. Oral antibiotic therapy is reserved for out-patient management, and if the patient is admitted into the hospital, then IV antibiotics are used. Complications may include: infertility, hydrosalpinx, adhesions, and Fitz-Hugh-Curtis syndrome, which consists of perihepatitis and fibrinous exudate with violin-string adhesions to anterior abdominal wall.

***Müllerian duct* fusion anomalies** include *uterine septum* and *uterine duplication*. Uterine *septum* may be *thin* or *thick*, or with poor vascular supply. The female internal genitals develop from the ***para**mesonephric (Müllerian) duct*. These include the formation of: the cervix, uterus, fallopian tubes, and the *upper* vagina. [Remember, although both male and females have paramesonephric and mesonephric ducts, when there is no Y chromosome the meso-nephric system will *regress*. The *male* internal genitals and Gartner's duct develop from the **mesonephric (Wolffian) duct.**]

## GARTNER'S DUCT CYSTS

These are *benign* cysts that are considered remnants of the *Wolffian* duct. They develop along the broad ligament down to the middle third of the vagina. Do NOT remove these cysts unless they are symptomatic.

# The Breast

---

## BREAST EXAMINATION

### SELF EXAMINATION
Self examination of the breast is recommended *monthly* for women over 20 years of age. By doing this, a woman may detect breast disease at an *early* stage. Self examination is usually done *after* the menstrual period, upright, with arms by the side, and then raised above the head. Palpate the supraclavicular and axillary lymph nodes and each breast quadrant with palmar side of the fingers and compress the nipples for any secretion. This is usually done while the individual is lying down.

### PHYSICIAN EXAMINATION
A physician exam of the breasts should be done at least once per year, checking for symmetry, and nipple or skin retraction—possible tumor growth beneath the surface, lymphadenopathy, and other changes. Palpation for any masses is usually done while the patient is upright, as well as in the supine position.

### MAMMOGRAPHY
This is a radiographic exam of the breasts used as a screening test and helpful in the diagnosis of a breast mass (it detects the smaller masses down to 1mm in diameter if there is calcification). The dose of radiation is very *low*, and the patient is under *low* risk for radiation exposure cancer. The American Cancer Society is a good source for breast mammography guidelines. It is recommended that the *baseline* mammogram be done from 35 to 40 years of age, and then each year or every 2 years from age 40 to 49 years. Women over 50 should have a mammography exam *each year*.

## NEOPLASM DIAGNOSIS

Pathologic lesions (any lump that is of question in the breast) are diagnosed by a 22-gauge *fine-needle aspiration biopsy or open breast biopsy*. Cytology will examine the aspirated tissue under histology. Then, you may excise the mass if necessary. (Fine-needle aspiration is NOT a definitive diagnosis.) Open breast biopsy is considered after the mammogram, fine-needle aspiration, family history, and clinical findings are assessed.

---

## LACTATION

The normal changes that allow lactation to occur in the breast include: breast *hypertrophy* during pregnancy, increased blood vessels and flow, and increased fat content. Lactation includes: *mammogenesis* (the growth and development of the breasts), *lactogenesis* (milk *secretion* with *prolactin* as the influencing hormone), and *galactopoiesis* (maintenance of milk secretion—by sucking and draining the milk; *oxytocin* is the influencing hormone that initiates milk *let-down*). Human milk is made of *water* (about 85 percent), sugar (*lactose*), fatty acids (*palmitic acid*), protein (casein and lactalbumin), enzymes (*amylase, lipase,* and others), immunoglobulins (mainly Ig**A**—which provides protection against bacteria), and leukocytes (monocytes, macrophages, and T and B cells).

---

## BENIGN BREAST DISEASE

### FIBROCYSTIC DISEASE OF THE BREAST

This is also known as *fibrocystic change disease*. This mammary dysplasia is the most common breast disease of women. It is present in approximately 50 percent of all women. Fibrocystic disease is most common among 20- to 40-year-old females (NOT postmenopausal women). It is associated with: cellular hyperplastic tissue changes of the breast (*hyperplasia*), *decreased* progesterone, and *increased* estrogen. Therefore, conditions *improve* during pregnancy (and lactation)—due to the increase in progesterone. Fibrocystic disease is characterized by: **bi**lateral, multiple *fibrous*-like lesions with premenstrual tenderness, and *pain*. Look for: *cysts* or *fibrosis* with or without epithelial cell *hyperplasia*, and *sclerosing adenosis* (intralobular fibrosis with proliferative epithelial ductules). There may be an increased risk of carcinoma; thus, you should check for a family history of breast carcinoma, and do a *baseline* mammography for any women over 25. Treatment includes: aspiration of the breast cyst to remove the fluid (also send it to cytology, especially if it is not clear fluid); avoidance of trauma by wearing support bras; analgesics; diuretics; Provera or progesterone may improve the symptoms.

### FIBROADENOMA

This is the most common *benign* breast tumor of women. It is associated with: a fibrous and glandular tissue tumor, and is usually a **uni**lateral, *freely mobile, solitary* growth (usually 1 to 10 cm; with the largest at up to a 15 cm diameter). The tumor usually grows during pregnancy and in the **pre**menopausal age group. Treatment includes: surgical excision (to verify that it is actually a benign fibroadenoma).

### GALACTOCELE
This is *cystic*, dilated ducts with thick, *milky* ("galacto") fluid. It is caused by obstruction of the duct by inflammation, infection, tumor, or fibrocystic disease. Treatment includes *fine-needle aspiration*. Anytime the aspirated fluid is *bloody*, it should be considered as possible breast cancer—biopsy is required.

### INTRADUCTAL PAPILLOMA
This is a ductal growth that usually occurs prior to or near *menopause*. It is usually in the lactiferous ducts. It is associated with: *bloody* or serous *discharge* from the nipple. Intraductal papillomas are considered *benign*, but may be *associated with* an increased risk of invasive breast carcinoma. They are the most common cause of bloody discharge from the nipple.

### PHYLLODES TUMOR
Also known as *cystosarcoma phyllodes*, this is a large tumor that may change the shape of the breast. It is usually a *benign* tumor, but may be a malignant tumor (rarely)—which may metastasize *hematogenously* to the lungs.

## MALIGNANT BREAST DISEASE

### CARCINOMA OF THE BREAST
Breast cancer is the most common malignancy in females. Risk factors include: positive family history, being over 40 years old (mean age of 60), **nulli**parity, *early* menarche, *late* menopause, increased dietary fat intake, and history of another carcinoma or radiation. Breast cancer spreads by the lymphatics or the blood system. *Axillary* lymph nodes are usually affected. *Hematogenous* spread usually occurs to the lungs and liver. The carcinoma is usually discovered as a lump by self examination or by a physician examination. Retraction or dimpling occurs as a result of skin involvement of the tumor mass. *Peau d'orange* is the *obstructed* skin *lymphatic* that leads to skin thickening. This will resemble an orange peel. Treatment includes the understanding of spread by hematogenous or lymphatic routes. Conservative surgery with radiation and/or chemotherapy may be indicated. (Oral contraceptives are NOT associated with an increase in the risk for breast cancer).

### THERAPIES FOR BREAST CANCER
*Radical mastectomy* includes: *en bloc* dissection of the entire breast, with the neighboring pectoralis major and minor, and the axillary node material. *Modified* radical mastectomy is usually the treatment used—*en bloc* removal of the breast and axillary lymph nodes, but NOT touching the pectoralis major muscle (just the fascia). Local radiation therapy with mastectomy can be used for patients with *negative* axillary nodes. *Partial* mastectomy is used in primary tumors that are small in size—local excision of the primary tumor.

Furthermore, reconstructive breast surgery may be offered to women who wish to regain their previous form—usually done after 3 months of surgery.

*Radiation therapy* may be given after excision of a tumor mass. Side effects may include: edema, soft tissue necrosis, and weakness.

*Chemotherapy* includes the combination therapy of the following drugs: **C**yclophosphamide, **M**ethotrexate, **A**driamycin (Doxorubicin), and 5-Fluorouracil. CMF is the usual combination used.

*Hormonal therapy* includes the understanding of estrogen receptor *positive* tumors. Anti-estrogen therapy includes Tamoxifen—which competes with estrogen for the estrogen receptors. Progesterone receptor–positive tumors also respond better to hormonal therapy. (The best response to hormonal therapy occurs in patients with *both* estrogen and progesterone receptor–positive tumors.)

Estrogen receptor *negative* tumors have the poorest prognosis—since the drugs cannot act on the receptors.

If a breast mass is found during pregnancy, the patient *should* receive a needle aspiration or open biopsy, and surgical treatment if necessary. Surgical treatment is usually NOT followed by irradiation. Chemotherapy has teratogenic risks. Therefore, a woman who is pregnant in the first trimester may consider abortion, and a pregnant woman in her third trimester may delay chemotherapy and then begin after delivery.

### INFILTRATING DUCTAL CARCINOMAS
These tumors make up the majority of breast cancers. Infiltrating or *invasive* breast cancer occurs as an *irregular*, *hard* nodule of 2 to 5 cm in size. It will appear on histologic exam as: anaplastic, large cells in cords, sheets or nests, in a *dense* stroma (which makes it a *hard nodule*).

#### Paget's disease of the breast
This is a form of intra**duct**al carcinoma of the large excretory ducts. It also affects the nipple and the areola as pruritis or eczematoid ulceration.

# Sexual Assault                    *10*

---

## RAPE

Rape is a violent attack or physical assault involving the *genitalia*, and a feeling of mutilation and death. Rape is sexual assault. Some women do not report sexual assault. They may appear calm, but have guilt, shame, and *fear*. *Power rape* is usually a *premeditated* assault imposed by a young male using *dominance*. *Anger rape* is usually an *impulsive* assault that often results in injury to the victim; the victim is often threatened with death if she reports the crime. *Sadistic rape* usually ends in *death* or *major injury*, and it is usually premeditated and the rapist is abusive.

In the examination of a rape victim, informed consent is taken for the exam and gathering of evidence. Documentation of an *alleged assault* must be recorded as to the physical injury, risks of pregnancy, assault history, location, and other factors. Remember, all health-care personnel should show respect and concern for the patient—to avoid additional emotional trauma. A thorough *pelvic examination* is necessary with a *witness* present, to check for abrasions and lacerations. Furthermore, photographs of the apparent injuries should be taken, and pubic hair samples (comb and cut, scrape under the fingernails). A pregnancy test should be performed and cultures should be taken of the blood (for VDRL), and an HIV test should be performed immediately and at a follow-up exam.

Treatment includes: treatment of any lacerations or injuries, *tetanus toxoid* to anyone who has not received a shot in the last 10 years, and STD prophylactic treatment (IM procaine penicillin and tetracycline—for syphilis, gonorrhea, trichomonas, and chlamydia risk). Furthermore, pregnancy issues may require drug contraception or first-trimester abortion. (NOTE: there is a risk when using *tetracycline*, which may retard bone growth and stain the teeth of the child.)

Follow-up care includes testing for gonorrhea (at 2 weeks), syphilis (at 6 weeks), and pregnancy testing. Also, the patient should have an appropriate (safe) living environment—to avoid another sexual assault.

If you are unable to provide adequate support as a physician, then you must refer professional help for the patient to adjust, and to decrease anxiety, and to treat depression, and other long-term psychological difficulties. As a physician, offer the patient care in a professional and compassionate manner.

# Reproductive Endocrinology

**11**

---
### FETUS

This is the *product of conception* (unborn) that occurs from the end of 8 weeks until birth.

---
### NEWBORN

This is otherwise known as the *neonate* and occurs from the time of birth through the first 28 days of life.

---
### INFANT

This is a baby *under* one year of age.

---
### CHILD

The time of *childhood* occurs between infancy and puberty. Childhood is often considered the time between 4 and 10 years old.

---
### PUBERTY

This is the time when the child is *transforming* into a young adult. It includes the production of gonadal hormones and secondary sexual characteristics. This follows from androgen production [like **d**eh**y**dro**e**pi**a**ndrosterone (DHEA)] from the *zona reticularis* (adrenal cortex). Puberty occurs at around the age of 12 for girls and 14 for boys.

---
### ADOLESCENT

An adolescent is an individual in the period between puberty and adulthood or maturity *(adolescence)*.

---

## PRECOCIOUS PUBERTY

This is the development of *secondary sexual characteristics* at an earlier age than the mean onset of puberty (about 8 to 9 years old). Usually the cause is idiopathic. The problem is that the long bone *epiphyses* will have premature fusion and this will lead to short stature. It is also associated with: virilizing tumor, congenital adrenal hyperplasia, and an ovarian tumor. About 90 percent of all female cases are *true precocious puberty*. These individuals have the onset of pulsatile GnRH, LH, and FSH release. In *pseudoisosexual precocious puberty*, there is an increase in estrogen or testosterone. This increased secretion may arise from ovarian tumors (granulosa-theca cell tumors), exogenous medications of cosmetics, or other functional tumor/cystic secretion.

Precocious puberty is diagnosed by physical examination, body weights and heights, and the *Tanner stages* of secondary sexual characteristics. Females with *masculinizing signs* and increased *androgens* are recommended to have a MRI or CT scan of the *adrenal glands*.

Treatment includes: GnRH analog treatment to suppress the release of LH and FSH and gonadotropin hormone; MPA, or medroxyprogesterone acetate; neurosurgery for tumor masses or CNS infections; and behavioral-psychosocial help. Check to make sure the patient isn't being exposed to *exogenous steroids*, and remove these from the environment if necessary. If the precocious puberty results from hypothyroidism, then supplement thyroid hormone. In *adrenal hyperplasia*, the glucocorticoids and mineralocorticoids are used.

---

## BREAST AND PUBIC HAIR DEVELOPMENT

*Marshall* and *Tanner* defined the stages of breast development and pubic hair development. The stages are simplified below:

| Stages of Breast Development |
| --- |
| 1   Preadolescent (elevated papilla) |
| 2   Breast *budding* |
| 3   Enlarging breast and areola (no separation) |
| 4   Projection of areola and papilla (above breast) |
| 5   *Mature* stage (recessed areola to breast level, projected papilla) |

| Stages of Pubic Hair Development |
| --- |
| 1   Preadolescent (no pubic hair) |
| 2   Sparse hair along the *labia* ("downy" hair) |
| 3   Spreading of hair (darker, coarser hair) |
| 4   Adult-type hair |
| 5   Adult-type hair with spreading to medial thighs ("inverse triangle" pattern) |

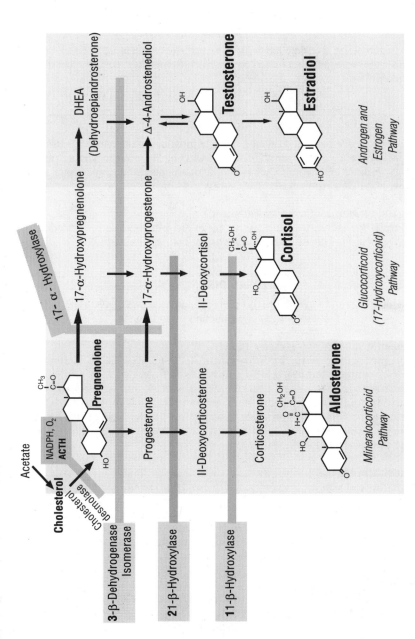

**Figure 11-1**  Steroid Synthesis Pathway

## VIRILISM

This occurs when a female has *masculine* somatic characteristics (deep voice, balding, clitoromegaly, increased coarse hair). Remember, *virile* means strong and masculine.

## HIRSUTISM

This is *excessive* body and facial *hair*. The most common cause of hirsutism is *heredity*, or a *positive family history*. Individuals from the Mediterranean race have more hirsutism. Other factors include: increased testosterone, idiopathic, and PCOD (polycystic ovarian disease).

### IDIOPATHIC HIRSUTISM (FAMILIAL HIRSUTISM)

If there is no increase in the androgen levels, but there is increased *hair* growth, then this is considered *idiopathic* or *familial* hirsutism.

## ADRENAL DISORDERS

Both hirsutism and virilism are the *signs* of increased *androgens*. The following may lead to the *adrenal gland* production of androgens.

### CONGENITAL ADRENAL HYPERPLASIA (CAH)

This is associated with: **21**-*hydroxylase* deficiency (with an increase in 17-hydroxyprogesterone), **11**-$\beta$-*hydroxylase* deficiency (with an increase in desoxycorticosterone and testosterone), *hirsutism*, and occasionally **3**-$\beta$-*hydroxysteroid dh* deficiency (with an increase in DHEA) (Fig. 11-1). Treatment includes glucocorticoids to correct for the deficient *cortisol*. CAH is the most common form of adrenal hyperplasia and is the most frequent cause of sexual ambiguity.

### CUSHING'S SYNDROME

This syndrome also leads to *increased androgen production* from *hypercortisolism*. Cushing's is due to a *cortisol*-producing tumor, increased ACTH production, and *increased adrenal gland function*. It is associated with: *moon-like face*, truncal *obesity*, abdominal *striae*, hirsutism, acne, hypertension, and *irregular* menses. Treat this condition by removing the ACTH or cortisol-producing tumor by surgical resection.

### CUSHING'S DISEASE

Cushing's *Disease* is Cushing's syndrome (increased ACTH) associated with a *pituitary basophil adenoma*—which results in increased adrenal function.

Again, it is characterized by an increased cortisol production by the *adrenal*. In Cushing's, we need to show an increased cortisol production, and an *inability to suppress* the secretion by dexamethasone. Low levels of ACTH suggests *adrenal adenoma* or a *carcinoma*. *High* levels of ACTH (or the inability to suppress the high-dose dexamethasone), suggests an ACTH-producing tumor.

**ADRENAL TUMORS**

These tumors, or adenomas, increase glucocorticoid (GC) and androgen production (like DHEA).

---

## OVARIAN DISORDERS

### POLYCYSTIC OVARIAN SYNDROME (PCOD)

This syndrome is also called **Stein-Levanthal Disease**, and includes: chronic *anovulation*, excessive *androgens*, *hirsutism* (PCOD is the most common cause of hirsutism among ovarian disorders), irregular menses, obesity, and infertility. The ovaries *and* the adrenal glands increase the secretion of androgens (with a normal ACTH level). Furthermore, the pituitary LH increases and this also increases the androgen production. Decreased FSH leads to chronic *anovulation*. The treatment includes estrogen-progesterone oral contraceptives.

### HYPERTHECOSIS

Stimulation of the ovarian leuteinizing stroma.

### OVARIAN TUMORS

Risk factors include a *positive family history* and **nulli**parity. They may occur in patients with late menopause. The *tumor marker*, or tumor-associated antigen **CA-125**, is used in detecting and documenting *ovarian cancer*. Neoplastic ovarian tumors include: epithelial, stromal, and germ-cell tumors.

#### Epithelial

These include: Brenner's tumor, epithelial tumors, serous or mucinous tumors, and endometrioid tumors. These tumors are derived from the *mesothelium* or *epithelium*.

##### SEROUS CYSTADENOMAS

Approximately 70 percent of serous cystadenomas are *benign*. They are usually **multi**locular and contain *psammoma bodies*.

##### MUCINOUS TUMOR

These are usually **multi**locular, **uni**lateral, and approximately 85 percent are *benign*.

##### BRENNER'S TUMOR

This is considered a relatively *benign* tumor (about 2 percent are malignant).

##### KRUKENBERG'S TUMOR

This is a malignant (metastatic) ovarian tumor from either the *gastrointestinal tract* or the *breast*. Remember, most Krukenberg's tumors are metastatic from the *stomach*, and they are usually **bi**lateral. Look for *signet-ring* cells on histologic exam of the tumor. Treat by removing the ovarian mass.

### Stromal

These include: sex-cord tumors, granulosa-theca tumors, Sertoli-Leydig tumors, and ovarian fibromas. Ovarian fibromas are associated with *Meig's syndrome* (ascites, hydrothorax, and ovarian fibroma). Most are found in *postmenopausal* women. Treatment includes: TAH and BSO in older women, or conservation of the uterus and contralateral ovary in young patients where a D&C shows no endometrial carcinoma.

#### GRANULOSA CELL TUMORS

Granulosa cell tumors are the most common *stromal* carcinomas. Check for the small grouping of cells or "Call-Exner bodies."

#### SERTOLI-LEYDIG CELL TUMORS

This tumor appears as a palpable mass, with an increase in androgens (like testosterone). These tumors are also called *arrhenoblastomas*.

#### LIPID CELL TUMORS

These *hilar cell tumors* are rare and occur in the ovary.

### Germ-cell tumors

Dysgerminoma and teratoma are the most common germ-cell tumors. The germ cell tumors produce human chorionic gonadotropin (hCG) or alpha-fetoprotein (AFP); therefore, hCG and AFP are considered *tumor markers*.

#### TERATOMA

This tumor includes multiple developmental tissues. It appears as a *benign* cystic tumor mass that may contain teeth, hair, and other tissues. (**Im**mature teratomas are considered *malignant*, and *mature* teratomas are considered *benign*.)

---

## TREATMENT OF HIRSUTISM

Estrogen-progestin oral contraceptive pills have been used in the treatment of hirsutism to decrease the gonadotropin production. This results in the decreased production of androgens (testosterone and androstenedione) by the ovaries. Congenital adrenal hyperplasia—Glucocorticoids (because of the low cortisol and negative feedback for ACTH). Cushing's syndrome—surgical removal of the producing tumor. (NOTE: Do NOT use oral contraceptives during pregnancy or in patients with deep vein thrombosis.)

#### SPIRONOLACTONE

This is an anti-androgen that acts as an *aldosterone antagonist*. It competes with aldosterone and testosterone, and it decreases the production of testosterone.

### COSMETICS AND LASER TECHNIQUES

Today, hirsutism is also treated *cosmetically* with shaving, electrolysis, and laser techniques. It is geared toward the removal of unwanted hair, and, if possible, the removal or depletion of the hair *follicles*.

## PRIMARY AMENORRHEA

This is defined as when there is NO spontaneous uterine bleeding through 16 and a half years old. The individual can only menstruate if she is given *exogenous* hormones. Furthermore, there may be no breast development (decreased estradiol secretion) and/or the individual may lack a uterus. Primary amenorrhea presents with the following breast and uterus conditions.

### HYPOGONADOTROPIC HYPOGONADISM

This is caused by hypothalamic or pituitary failure. A *lower* FSH level suggests **hypo**gonadotropic hypogonadism, and an *increased* FSH suggests *gonadal dysgenesis* (LH and estradiol levels do NOT help us in diagnosis).

Performing a GnRH test (although not really that helpful) will differentiate if the hypogonadotropic hypogonadism is from a *hypothalamic* or a *pituitary* origin. Giving exogenous GnRH should have a LH response—if there is **no** response, this is probably from a *pituitary failure*.

### HYPERGONADOTROPIC HYPOGONADISM

A genetic or enzyme (hydroxylase) deficiency can cause *gonadal dysgenesis*. This causes **hyper**gonadotropic hypogonadism and NO gonadal development. Consider Turner's syndrome (45 XO), abnormal X chromosome, 17-hydroxylase deficiency, and other disorders affecting the X chromosome or an added Y chromosome. These patients are *sterile*. Treatment includes estrogen-progestin supplements. This will assist second sexual characteristics (breast development).

### ANDROGEN INSENSITIVITY SYNDROME

This includes *testicular feminization syndrome* where the *phenotypical* females have *testicles*. The testosterone level is in the normal range for a *male*. Therefore, it is necessary to *karyotype* these patients. Treatment includes removal of the testicles ("gonads") to prevent tumors, and medical estrogen replacement.

### CONGENITAL ABSENCE OF THE UTERUS

These patients lack a uterus, but have ovaries. The testosterone level is in the normal range for a *female*.

## SECONDARY AMENORRHEA

This is *amenorrhea* (no menses) for at least 6 months, when the individual had *regular* menses in the past—or amenorrhea for one year if the patient had *oligomenorrhea*.

First, check to make sure the patient is not pregnant. Then, consider any drugs, stress, or weight changes that may relate to the amenorrhea. Then, note the estrogen (*low* levels = NO bleeding), FSH, and LH levels. If history warrants, identify if there are any *uterine adhesions* by scope.

### Hypothalamic dysfunction
This may occur in patients with stress, weight changes, or drugs. The serum LH will be *normal*. Treatment may include: correct the etiologic factor (like stress) and if the estrogen level is low, consider estrogen replacement.

### Hypothalamic-pituitary failure
This is associated with a *low* FSH level. Causes include: anorexia nervosa (*severe* weight loss), Sheehan's syndrome (*low* prolactin level), pituitary adenoma, and hypothalamic lesions. Treatment may include: gonadotropins or estrogen-progestin replacement, or surgery to remove a pituitary mass.

### Premature ovarian failure
This is associated with a *high* FSH level.

## HYPERPROLACTINEMIA

Hyperprolactinemia is associated with *causing* oligomenorrhea, amenorrhea, and galactorrhea. The *increase* in *prolactin* level may be caused by drugs like TCAs, antihypertensives, and narcotics—decreasing the catecholamines. Remember, dopamine normally *inhibits* prolactin. Therefore, if the dopamine *decreases*, then the prolactin will *increase*. Etiologic factors of hyperprolactinemia (*high* prolactin level) include: **hypo**thyroidism (*low* $T_4$ and dopamine *increases* the TSH and *prolactin*), prolactin-secreting *pituitary adenomas*, craniopharyngioma (non-pituitary tumor), and acromegaly.

Treatment includes *discontinuing* any causative medication, observation, bromocriptine (a dopamine agonist), given to *inhibit* pituitary secretion of prolactin and *increase* estrogen secretion, discontinuing lactation, and *transsphenoidal* surgical removal of a pituitary adenoma. Treat hypothyroidism with thyroid hormone replacement therapy.

### Galactorrhea
This is continuous milk discharge from the breast (with NO pus or blood), and usually occurring **bi**laterally.

## INFERTILITY

A couple is considered *infertile* when they are unsuccessful in conceiving after 6 to 12 months of unprotected intercourse. In order to conceive, the two individuals who have reported this failure will need to be evaluated. Factors include: age (women over 35), factors of sexual intercourse (frequency and timing), tubal patency, cervical mucus pH (best above 6.5), history of exces-

| Menstruation | |
| --- | --- |
| Normal menstruation | Normal bleeding every 21 to 35 days (menstrual period for 1 to 5 days). |
| **Abnormal Uterine Bleeding** | |
| **(When the frequency or intensity of the uterine bleeding changes)** | |
| Metrorrhagia | Intermenstrual bleeding, or bleeding that occurs *between* periods. |
| Menometrorrhagia | Irregular *frequency* of bleeding and *increased* amount. |
| Hypermenorrhea | This is a cyclic or regular bleeding, but in *increased* amount or duration. |
| Hypomenorrhea | *Decreased* menstrual flow ("spotting"), this can occur with oral contraceptive use. |
| Oligomenorrhea | Varying bleeding that occurs in intervals longer than 35 days. "Scanty" menstruation. This can occur in anovulatory cycles. |
| Polymenorrhea | Vaginal bleeding that occurs *more* than every 21 days. |
| Postmenopausal bleeding | Vaginal bleeding that happens after **1** year since LMP of menopausal woman. |
| Breakthrough bleeding | Bleeding during estrogen stimulation, with no decrease in the estrogen levels. |
| **Additional Alterations** | |
| Dysmenorrhea | Difficult and *painful* menstruation, menstrual "cramps." |
| Mittelschmerz | Midcycle (intermenstrual) pain, abdominal pain around the time of *ovulation*. |
| Dyspareunia | Pain during sexual intercourse. |

sive alcohol intake, Basal Body Temperature (BBT should be elevated 0.5 to 0.8°F for at least 11 days during the luteal phase), smoke or other environmental exposure, male history of *mumps orchitis* or other genital tract infections, inadequate testosterone production, semen analysis (form, volume, motility, maturity, or increased leukocytes), and endocrine problems (thyroid problems and increased FSH).

Therapy for infertility should be directed toward improving all factors.

Semen analysis requires the male to have 2 to 3 days without ejaculation, and to assess an ejaculation specimen within 1 h. The semen should be 2 to 5 ml in volume, over 20 million/ml sperm count, with over 50 percent sperm motility and a pH of 7.2 to 7.8. A repeat test is done a week later. Risk factors for abnormal sperm include: smoking, alcohol intake, environmental hazards, epididymitis, and increased temperature of the scrotum.

## OVULATION

Basal body temperature or BBT is a relatively abandoned test to evaluate ovulation but, because it has been seen to show up on your exams, you may want to be familiar with it. The temperature is taken in the *morning* prior to any work. A luteal phase defect is associated with: irregular cervical mucus, non-rising BBT, previous history of a *spontaneous abortion*, and *endometriosis*. Medications, like *Clomiphene*—an anti-estrogen that increases the FSH, but may increase the risk of multiple births—or *progesterone supplementation*, are used in treating this luteal phase defect. "Predictor kits" may also be used for a good estimate of ovulation.

## ANATOMICAL FACTORS

Uterine anatomical factors may affect the ability to impregnate (see Fig. 11-2). Endometrial polyps, *endometriosis*, prior salpingitis (or infection), previous IUD use, and other forms of occlusion (most commonly in the *isthmus near the*

**Uterus Subseptus Unicollis**

**Uterus Septus Duplex**

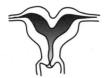

**Uterus Bicornis Unicollis (U.B.U.)**

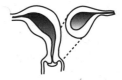

**U.B.U. with an
unconnected rudimentary horn**

**Figure 11-2**   Uterine Anomalies

*cornu*). Endometriosis may obstruct the fallopian tube and the motility, and cause adhesions. Physical examination, hysterosalpingography (HSG), laparoscopy, and radiography are used to diagnose anatomical disruptions. These anatomical obstructions may be treated by *microsurgical tuboplasty* for reanastomosis or may need to be bypassed by in vitro fertilization.

## ENDOMETRIOSIS

This is the presence of *ectopic* endometrial tissue that may appear as cystic masses of blood. Endometriosis is a *benign* condition where the endometrial tissue appears *outside* of the endometrial cavity. The most common site of endometriosis is in the *ovary* (although other sites are associated with *infertility*), and it can also occur in the pelvic peritoneum, the broad ligament, rectovaginal septum, and the colon. An ovarian *endometrioma* forms and contains a *chocolate-colored fluid*–filled cyst (hemolyzed blood).

The triad of symptoms includes: (1) *Dysmenorrhea* (painful/difficult menstruation), (2) *Dyspareunia* (pain during intercourse), and (3) *Dyschezia* (difficulty in defecation). Protein C3 (blood coagulation factor) is present in the endometrial glands, and the patient may have an abnormal autoimmune function. Endometriosis occurs bilaterally. The benign glands invade gastrointestinal and genitourinary organs. Look for these other signs on physical examination: on ultrasound—firm, tender adnexal mass; ESR and wbc are within normal limits, but there is an increase in CA-125.

Endometriosis is associated with nulliparous women in their thirties. *Laparoscopy* gives a definitive diagnosis.

Medical management includes: hormonal therapy (Provera), Danazol (if fertility is not a concern), oral contraceptives, and GnRH analogs (Lupron and Nafarelin). Women over 40 may be treated with surgery: check with fractional D&C and rule out endometrial carcinoma; surgical resection, total abdominal hysterectomy (TAH), and bilateral salpingo-oophorectomy (BSO); and the use of laser surgery or photocoagulation. *In vitro* fertilization may be necessary for fertilization of a patient with endometriosis.

## INCOMPETENT CERVIX

This is a dilated cervix that results in prolapse and rupture of the membrane. This will induce the discharge of a non-viable fetus.

## MENOPAUSE

Menopause is the time of *permanent cessation of menses*; the time after the LMP or last menstrual period (NOT a sudden loss of function of the ovary—it is *gradual* with *anovulation* and irregular cycles). Menopause occurs from 50 to 55 years of age. The woman no longer makes enough estrogen to prepare the tissue. Remember, women are born with approximately 1,500,000 ova, and over the years they will end up with approximately one third or

400,000 ova. This is because they will use the *responsive ova* in the nearly four decades of menstruation.

After the remaining ova are occluded the ovary does not respond and the *hormone production decreases*. These hormones affect distant organs (as well as the ovary), and this leads to changes in the body tissues. The low hormone levels (of estrogen, and progesterone) lead to the various physical changes including: calcium loss in bone tissue, decreased collagen in skin, "hot flashes," insomnia, and neurologic changes. These sex-hormone related problems may lead to disability in some women. The "hot flashes" are thought to be due to the decrease in estrogen, which alerts the *hypothalamus* to release GnRH (gonadotropin *releasing* hormone)—to finally increase the *anterior pituitary* "pulsatile" release of FSH and LH.

The most common problem in post-menopausal women is *osteoporosis*, and this results in *compression fractures*.

For this reason, women are encouraged to consider *estrogen* (oral Premarin) and *progesterone replacement therapy* (progestogen or Provera). In a hysterectomized woman, give only *estrogen* replacement therapy.

# Obstetric and Gynecologic Procedures

---

## 12

## DILATATION AND CURETTAGE (D&C)

This is the most common *gynecologic surgical procedure*. It includes the *dilatation* of the *cervix*, and then the *curettage* of the *endometrium*. It is used for determining cancer of the cervix or endometrium, and can be *diagnostic* as well as *therapeutic*. D&Cs are performed for: irregular *menstrual bleeding*, irregular endometrial cavity, endometrial polyps, and first-trimester pregnancies. Complications include: *hemorrhage*, infection, laceration of the cervix, and *perforated uterus*.

---

## HYSTERECTOMY

This is a common surgical procedure. An *abdominal* hysterectomy is performed for removing the corpus, cervix, and/or the uterus with tissue and ligaments. This procedure is indicated in: benign fibroids, chronic PID, and some malignant diseases of the cervix, ovary and endometrium. A *vaginal* hysterectomy will avoid an abdominal scar. This is done when the uterus is mobile, not that large, and there are NO adhesions. It is indicated in: uterine prolapse and CIN (carcinoma *in situ*).

A colposcopy may be required to rule out cervical carcinoma. The most serious complication of a hysterectomy is *injury* to the *ureter*—lateral to the cervix or under the infundibulopelvic ligament. The patient will present with flank pain and a fever. On an exam and in practice, this is important to remember. Be careful of the ureter! Also, other complications, like atelectasis, infection (pelvic cellulitis), UTI, and pulmonary embolism may occur.

---

## LAPAROSCOPY

This is the use of a *laparoscope* to view the *peritoneal cavity*. It can be used in evaluating *infertility*, pelvic masses, and is therapeutic for *tubal sterilization*. A *laparoscopy* is performed to find, by *scope*, an ovarian *cyst* in a patient with a large adrenal mass and severe pelvic pain. Laparoscopy is *contraindicated* in bowel obstruction.

## COLPOSCOPY

Using a *colposcope* (a type of stereoscopic microscope), a speculum is placed to view the *cervix*, cleaning the area (with 3% acetic acid-soaked cotton). The squamous epithelium (grayish color), and the columnar epithelium (reddish color) can be identified. The *cervical dysplasia* or a *condyloma* can be biopsied, and vascular differences can be seen.

## AMNIOCENTESIS

This is a prenatal diagnostic test to withdraw amniotic fluid from the sac. It is used in checking for chromosomal abnormalities and neural tube defects. Do an *ultrasound-guided* amniocentesis at 16 to 20 weeks.

## CHORIONIC VILLOUS SAMPLING (CVS)

This checks for chromosomal, enzyme, and biochemical abnormalities, and is usually done at 9 to 12 weeks. (It CANNOT measure AFP.)

## CORDOCENTESIS

This is percutaneous umbilical blood sampling (blood from the *umbilical* vein), and is done at 10 to 22 weeks to assist in evaluation of genetic disease and obstetric complications.

## ULTRASOUND

This uses sound waves to determine *structural abnormalities* of the fetus that may have been exposed to teratogenic agents, has defects, or has been exposed to the diabetes mellitus of the mother, affecting an increase in heart or skeletal defects. A *pelvic ultrasound* is preferred during *laparotomy of a cyst* from an ovary (cystectomy) over laparoscope.

## PAPANICOLAOU TEST

The Papanicolaou test (smear) will detect preinvasive cervical cancer. The atypical squamous metaplasia occurs in the transformation zone, and causes a change, cervical intraepithelial neoplasia (CIN). CIN is the preinvasive phase of cervical carcinoma. The "Pap smear" is recommended as an annual exam after a woman has become sexually active. Histologic samples are taken from the *endocervical canal* and the *ectocervix*. The Pap smear will detect an abnormal cervix (*squamous* cervical lesions cover the columnar epithelium).

In a patient with *severe dysplasia*, the next step after a *Pap smear* should be *colposcopy* with *direct biopsy*. If there is a *gross lesion*, the next step is to *biopsy* (there is no need for colposcopy).

---

## TOLUIDINE BLUE

Biologic stain used after a hysterectomy if there may be leakage in urine (reddish color). If there is NO toluidine blue then it can be considered a *ureterovaginal fistula*.

---

## REGIONAL ANALGESIC AND ANESTHETIC TECHNIQUES

### EPIDURAL ANALGESIA

This gives *excellent* anesthesia during labor in a vaginal delivery. An *epidural* is given as *continuous* lumbar analgesia between the **L3** to **L4** levels, during labor when the cervix is 4 to 5 cm in multiparous women or 5 to 6 in nulliparous women, and when there are strong uterine contractions. It allows for analgesia at levels **T10** to **L1**, to decrease the pain from the *uterus* (from the *visceral* **a**fferent nerves). An initial small test dose is given, and if there is *tachycardia*, then you made an IV injection error! Medications include small doses of local anesthetic (bupivacaine). IV crystalloid solution is given to prevent *hypotension*.

### PARACERVICAL BLOCK

A *paracervical block* anesthetizes the *sensory* nerves of the uterus at the **T10** to **L1** levels. A transvaginal injection is made with local anesthetic *bilaterally* to the cervix. It *is* associated with fetal distress and may cause maternal toxicity. (It is NOT associated with maternal hypotension.)

### SPINAL BLOCK

Also called a *subarachnoid block*, it is given right before delivery. Using a spinal needle at the **L3-L4** interspace, give a small dose injection of local anesthetic (like lidocaine, or bupivacaine) with 10% dextrose in the sitting position. IV crystalloid solution is given to prevent *hypotension*. The patient may experience a *headache* after delivery.

### PUDENDAL BLOCK

A *pudendal block* anesthetizes the *pudendal* nerve at the **S2** to **S4** levels. Given just prior to delivery, it allows *perineal analgesia* for vaginal delivery. This allows the mother to have analgesia for a low-forceps delivery and episiotomy (*perineal* pain—from *somatic* **a**fferent nerves). (It usually does NOT cause fetal distress, and is NOT associated with maternal hypotension.)

# *Abortion* 13

NOTE: *Although we discussed abortion in Chaps. 4 and 5, this short chapter is provided as a review of many tested areas that are important for you to understand. Repetition is provided for your increased understanding of this material.*

## ABORTION

*Abortion* is the *unplanned* or spontaneous loss of a pregnancy (fetus or embryo) during fetal development—at a time when the fetus is **un**able to survive if it is outside of the mother's womb. (*Termination of pregnancy* is the *purposeful* discontinuance of pregnancy.) Spontaneous abortions occur often, but the cause is still difficult to assess. Some factors that may increase the likelihood of an abortion include: *fetal genetic abnormality* (this is the body's natural defense mechanism to abort a fetus with chromosomal anomalies), infections (*Listeria monocytogenes, Syphilis, Toxoplasma or CMV*), psychological influences and sudden changes to the body, environmental toxins, teratogenic drugs, smoking, alcoholic consumption, uterine abnormalities and medical disorders (SLE, DM, and hypothyroidism), increased maternal age, and possible paternal chromosomal abnormalities.

## β-HCG

The level of β-**h**uman **c**horionic **g**onadotropin should be measured during a suspected pregnancy. It rises after 7 to 10 days from the date of conception, and offers an estimate for the gestational age. The increase occurs approximately 9 days after the midcycle LH surge (ovulation), and peaks at approximately 60 to 90 days. It then assists in the maintenance of the progesterone and corpus luteum. Spontaneous abortion occurs in up to 50 percent of all pregnancies—with the majority in the first 2 weeks. Increased maternal age will increase the risk for an abortion (significant rise after 40 years of age). The hCG doubling time is 48 hours.

## THREATENED ABORTION

A pregnancy (viable embryo) is "threatened" when there is a complication of *vaginal bleeding* before week 20. It is associated with: *closed* internal cervical os, vaginal *bleeding*, *abdominal ache* (mild cramping, NOT pain), but NO fever. Many *threatened* abortions will ultimately abort. But remember, many women will have vaginal bleeding during the first trimester of pregnancy. An ultrasound exam is done to determine if the fetus is alive (about 95 percent of the live fetuses will go on to a live birth). Repeat the ultrasound exam in a week to reassure the patient that the fetus is well.

## INEVITABLE ABORTION

This is a pregnancy that is associated with *heavy* vaginal *bleeding*, abdominal *pain*, and partially dilated cervix (opened internal os)—leading to an "inevitable" abortion. These patients need to be *admitted to the hospital* for an emergency D & C. Also, perform an ultrasound exam.

## MISSED ABORTION

This is a "missed" abortion because the fetus is dead (there is NO viable embryo), and it remained in the uterus—possibly for a few weeks. A missed abortion does NOT have bleeding, cramping, fever, or any passed tissue. Perform an ultrasound exam, then if necessary, evacuate the products of conception.

## INCOMPLETE ABORTION

This is associated with: vaginal *bleeding*, abdominal *pain*, cervical dilation, and secretion of clumpy *parts* of the products of conception. These patients need to be *admitted to the hospital*, then insert an IV line and type and cross the blood—to be ready for hemorrhage or infection causing shock. Treat with an emergency D & C. Incomplete abortions may lead to an overwhelming sepsis and DIC.

## COMPLETE ABORTION

This is associated with: secretion of *all* of the products of conception, *closure* of the cervix, *negative* pregnancy test, and minimal to no bleeding. These patients should be observed and you must rule out an *ectopic pregnancy* by transvaginal sonography.

## SEPTIC ABORTION

This is associated with: secretion of the products of conception, *varied* bleeding and abdominal cramping, cervical dilation, and *FEVER*.

## SURGICAL METHODS OF ABORTION

### VAGINAL EVACUATION

Two techniques are used in the vaginal evacuation of a pregnancy. *Suction curettage* and *Dilatation & Curettage* (D & C). Suction is more rapid (less than 5 minutes), has a decreased need for cervical dilation (fewer cervical lacerations), and anesthesia (less pain), and produces better results with less trauma and infection.

### DILATATION & CURETTAGE (D & C)

D & C is done to diagnose irregular or heavy menstrual bleeding and post-menopausal bleeding. It can be therapeutic for removing the products of conception following an abortion. The dilatation of the cervix and the curettage of the endometrium is actually the most common surgical procedure in gynecology. It is done to determine if *endometrial* or *cervical cancer* is present in the strips of tissue. The *myometrium* is the stopping area—when you get to a grinding feeling in the curettage procedure. Remember, a D & C is performed on *missed, inevitable,* and *incomplete* abortions. Complications include: *hemorrhage,* infection, laceration of the cervix, and perforation of the uterus.

### INDUCTION OF CONTRACTIONS

Induction of uterine contractions is done by infusing *intraamniotic saline,* and *prostaglandin* ($PGF_2$ or $PGE_2$ *Prostin*)—intraamniotic, intravaginal suppositories, or intramuscular. Prostaglandins cause vasospasms.

### COMPLICATIONS OF AN INDUCED ABORTION

Induced abortion methods include: menstrual extraction, suction and sharp curettage, dilation and evacuation, induction of labor by amniotic infusion (or vaginal suppositories), and hysterotomy/hysterectomy. The complications include: failed termination, perforated uterus, hemorrhage, infection, cervical laceration, emotional stress, and embolism. Morbidity worsens with second trimester abortions (compared to first). Remember, the increased *number of weeks* gestation *increases* the maternal morbidity and mortality. Also, a *hysterectomy* procedure has the highest maternal mortality rate (approximately 25/100,000), while suction curettage has a low maternal mortality rate (approximately 1/100,000). (See Table 5-1.)

## TERMINATION OF PREGNANCY

The legal limit of gestational age of termination, and the conditions of the pregnancy are factors in terminating pregnancy. Dilation of the cervix and the aspiration curettage under paracervical block or general anesthesia is the procedure for *first* trimester termination. RU-486 is a drug that has been used in the first trimester to terminate pregnancy. This *anti-progesterone medication* is also given with *prostaglandins*. *Second* trimester termination of pregnancy (usually due to a genetic deformity) is induced by *prostaglandins*. The dilatation and evacuation of the fetus and placental parts will decrease the painful process from the medical termination.

## RU 486

This medication is an *antiprogestin* that is used to offer *postcoital* contraception by *interrupting the implantation*.

# Additional Concepts about Female Cancers

**14**

The number one cancer is *breast cancer*, followed by colorectal, lung, endometrial, and ovarian cancer.

## BREAST CANCER

This is the most common female malignancy. It will occur in approximately 1 out of 12 women. The risk factors include: positive family history, **nulli-parity**, *early* menarche, *late* menopause, being over forty years of age, increased fat consumption, obesity, other cancers, fibrocystic change with *atypia*, and previous radiation.

### INFILTRATING DUCT CARCINOMA
**Paget's disease** is an intraductal carcinoma which appears in the nipple and the areola. The treatment is *radical mastectomy* to dissect the breast, pectoralis major and minor, and the axillary contents. A *modified* radical mastectomy leaves the muscles intact, and is augmented by radiation and combination chemotherapy—Cyclophosphamide, MTX, 5-FU, and Doxorubicin (Adriamycin).

## CIN, OR CERVICAL INTRAEPITHELIAL NEOPLASIA

There are NO signs or symptoms for CIN. Again, there are NO signs or symptoms for CIN. Remember, most cancers are **a**symptomatic. With CIN III, do a *colposcopy* with direct *biopsy*.

## GESTATIONAL TROPHOBLASTIC NEOPLASIA

This includes: *benign hydatidiform moles*, and two malignant forms—*invasive mole* and *choriocarcinoma*. The tumor marker to evaluate GTN is an increased secretion from the tumor of $\beta$**-hCG**. Incidence is 1 in 1500 to 2000 pregnancies with an increase in Asian women (Far East

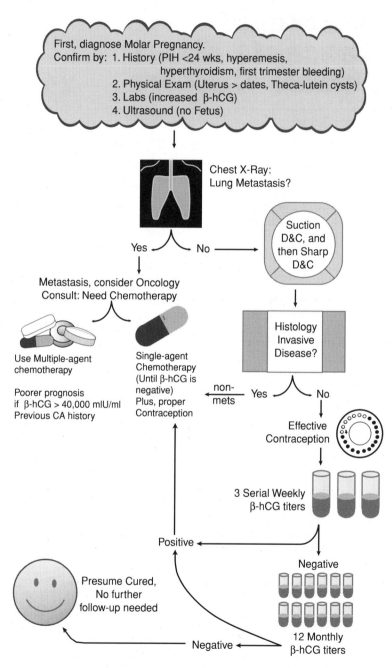

First, diagnose Molar Pregnancy.
Confirm by: 1. History (PIH <24 wks, hyperemesis,
hyperthyroidism, first trimester bleeding)
2. Physical Exam (Uterus > dates, Theca-lutein cysts)
3. Labs (increased β-hCG)
4. Ultrasound (no Fetus)

Chest X-Ray:
Lung Metastasis?

Yes    No

Suction
D&C, and
then Sharp
D&C

Metastasis, consider Oncology
Consult: Need Chemotherapy

Use Multiple-agent
chemotherapy

Poorer prognosis
if β-hCG > 40,000 mIU/ml
Previous CA history

Single-agent
Chemotherapy
(Until β-hCG is
negative)
Plus, proper
Contraception

Histology
Invasive
Disease?

non-
mets    Yes    No

Effective
Contraception

3 Serial Weekly
β-hCG titers

Positive

Negative

Presume Cured,
No further
follow-up needed

Negative    12 Monthly
β-hCG titers

**Figure 14-1**  Management of Molar Pregnancy

Asians > Asian Americans). GTN has been associated in areas with a *decreased* consumption of *folic acid* and *β-carotene.*

### HYDATIDIFORM MOLE

During the first and the beginning of second trimester, the patient presents with irregular and *heavy* (but, usually *painless*) vaginal *bleeding*, and lower abdominal pain. This occurs with hyperemesis and *hypertension.* The signs may appear as: similar to *hyperthyroidism* (increased heart rate, hypertension, and tachypnea), absent fetal heart sounds, and pre-eclampsia. The β-hCG titers may be extremely *high* in the early trimesters, which may suggest possible *gestational trophoblastic neoplasia* or *multiple* gestation. An *ultrasound* will show a *"snow-storm"* pattern.

The majority of hydatidiform moles are *complete* and will appear as a *bunch of grapes.* They usually have a **46 XX** karyotype and both X chromosomes are *paternal.*

Treatment includes: *suction evacuation* and *sharp curretage* of the uterus. Oxytocin will decrease the amount of blood loss and increase the uterine contractions. After the evacuation of the molar pregnancy, you must *follow the β-hCG titers* to make certain there is a decline over the next three months (see Fig. 14-1). It is important that the patient does not become pregnant for at least one year—so that the titers can be followed appropriately.

A *partial* or incomplete mole presents with a *coexistent fetus* as a spontaneous or missed abortion. These moles usually have a *triploid* karyotype or **69 XXY.**

### INVASIVE MOLE

This is an invasive malignant mole that may enter the myometrium or uterus and cause hemorrhage. β-hCG titers tend to remain high even after an evacuation. Treat with *hysterectomy.* Invasive moles are usually NOT associated with metastases.

### CHORIOCARCINOMA

This is a *malignant* GTN, and can display hematogenous spread to the lungs, vagina, brain, and GI tract. It appears as: *vaginal bleeding, hemoptysis* (with lung involvement), dizziness (brain metastasis), and GI bleeding (GI metastasis). Chemotherapy includes: (MAC) **M**ethotrexate, **A**ctinomycin-D, and **C**yclophosphamide; or other combinations of anti-cancer medications. Follow the β-hCG titers during treatment.

---

## CERVICAL CANCER

Cancer of the cervix is usually found in women over the age of 47 years. Cervical intraepithelial neoplasia (CIN) is associated with **H**uman **P**apilloma **V**irus (HPV) types 16, 18, 31, 33, and 35. (HPV types 6 and 11 are associated with *cervical condylomata.*) The Pap smear is done to check changes in the cervical epithelium or the normal *columnar* to the *squamous* vaginal epithelium. Patients do NOT present with *symptoms.* A *colposcopy* is performed for symptoms of *painless* vaginal bleeding, and cryosurgery of the transformation zone, or hysterectomy and radiation for CIN III. The standard staging system was designed by the *International Federation of Gynecology and Obstetrics (FIGO)*.

The stages of CIN and the affected areas are:

| | |
|---|---|
| 0 | Carcinoma *in situ* (CIS)—this is considered *preinvasive* |
| I | Cervix only |
| II | Beyond cervix and upper ⅔ of vagina |
| III | Cervix to the lower ⅓ of vagina, and the pelvic wall |
| IV | Beyond the pelvis |
| | (**IVa** is spread to *adjacent* organs; **IVb** to *distant* organs) |

## OVARIAN CANCER

The risk of ovarian cancer increases with *nulliparous* women. The standard staging system was designed by *FIGO*.

The general stages of ovarian cancer and the affected areas are:

| | |
|---|---|
| I | Unilateral or bilateral ovaries *only* |
| II | Ovaries and pelvis to uterus |
| III | Ovaries and peritoneal implants |
| IV | Ovaries and distant metastasis |

### OVARIAN NEOPLASMS

#### 1. Epithelial
Multilocular serous cystadenoma, psammoma bodies in serous tumors ("sand," calcific). Brenner tumor is a large, solid, *benign*, mucinous epithelial tumor.

#### 2. Stromal
Sex cord-stromal ovarian neoplasms, fibromas, granulosa-thecal cell tumors, or Sertoli-Leydig cell tumors occur from the *sex cords*. Ovarian fibroma is a nonfunctioning neoplasm that produces NO secretions. *Meigs' syndrome* includes: *ascites*, right *hydrothorax*, with an *ovarian fibroma*.

#### 3. Germ-cell
These neoplasms occur at any age, and compose approximately 60 percent of ovarian neoplasms. The most common *benign* germ-cell tumor is a hair- or sebaceous-filled dermoid cyst (benign *cystic teratoma* of a germ cell origin.)

#### 4. Mixed cell

Management: Epithelial ovarian neoplasms need *unilateral salpingo-oophorectomy*, and there is an increase in malignancy in the bilateral and serous tumors. Stromal-cell tumors also need *salpingo-oophorectomy* and germ-cell tumors are managed by *ovarian cystectomy.*

---

## VULVAR AND VAGINAL CANCER

Approximately 90 percent of vulvar cancers are *squamous cell carcinomas.* *Malignant melanoma* that affects the clitoris or labia minora comprises the second most common type of vulvar cancer. These cancers increase in postmenopausal women over the age of 65 who are obese, and have hypertension or diabetes. In diagnosing lower genital tract lesions, you should perform a *punch biopsy* if there is a lesion in question. If the patient has itching in the vulva (*vulvar pruritus*), but there is NO lesion, then use colposcopy to find a good site to *biopsy.* This is especially true for a postmenopausal woman around 65 years old with a history of *chronic vulvar itching*—you should think of possible *squamous cell carcinoma of the vulva.* Diethylsylbesterol (DES) is associated with *clear-cell adenocarcinoma* of the *vagina* in the female offspring of the mother who took this medication. The staging for vulvar cancer is based on the *FIGO* Cancer Committee surgical staging system.

The stages of vulvar carcinoma include:

| | |
|---|---|
| 0 | Carcinoma *in situ* (CIS) |
| I | Vulva affected, ≤2 cm, no lymph node metastasis |
| II | Vulva and/or perineum, >2 cm, no lymph node |
| III | Adjacent spread to urethra and/or vagina or anus, **uni**lateral lymph node metastasis |
| IV | IVa = Invasion |
| | IVb = Distant metastasis |

### FIBROMA OF THE VULVA
This is a manifestation of von Recklinghausen's disease and is treated by surgical removal.

### BARTHOLIN'S CYST
This is the most common vulvar tumor. Usually, it appears as a unilateral mass that occurs secondary to an infection—which produces an abscess. The treatment includes marsupialization of the gland with a fistulous tract to the skin.

Treatment for vulvar carcinoma is directed to follow *local excision* of the lesions (NOT total vulvectomy), and laser therapy. Medical treatment includes topical 5-fluorouracil cream.

## ENDOMETRIAL CARCINOMA

The inner membrane layer of the uterine wall (endometrium) creates abnormal vaginal *bleeding*. It is associated with the elderly, obese, or hypertensive patient. It is diagnosed with *laparoscopy*. The treatment is an *exploratory laparotomy* with adjuvant radiation or modified radical hysterectomy with BSO. The stages of endometrial carcinoma are:

| | |
|---|---|
| 0 | Carcinoma *in situ* (CIS) |
| I | Carcinoma of the corpus |
| II | Carcinoma of the corpus and cervix |
| III | Outside the uterus (not the pelvis) |
| IV | Outside the pelvis |
| | **IVa** spreads to *adjacent* organs |
| | **IVb** spreads to *distant* organs |

### ENDOMETRIAL POLYPS

These are a form of myoma, cancer, carcinosarcoma, or polypoid endometrial hyperplasia. Only 5 percent are considered malignant, and they are associated with *postmenopausal* women and abnormal *bleeding*.

## ENDOMETRIAL HYPERPLASIA

This is an increased growth of endometrium, with increased estrogen and no progesterone. It presents as: post-menopausal *bleeding* or irregular and prolonged menstrual bleeding with clots, anemia, and an *enlarged uterus*. Treatment includes Provera for a younger patient (medroxyprogesterone acetate) and for heavy bleeding consider a D&C. If it recurs, then consider progestogens or a hysterectomy. The variants of endometrial hyperplasia include:

### CYSTIC GLANDULAR HYPERPLASIA

It possesses a "Swiss cheese" microscopic pattern and is a precursor of endometrial cancer.

### ADENOMATOUS HYPERPLASIA

These glands are not cystic and the stroma does NOT participate in hyperplastic reaction. The more cellular atypia and cytologic changes increase the chance of endometrial CA.

| Cancer/Syndrome | Marker |
|---|---|
| Embryonal carcinoma | Increased level of β-hCG and AFP |
| Gestational Trophoblastic Neoplasia (*invasive* mole and *choriocarcinoma*) | Increased level of β-hCG |
| Endodermal sinus tumor Neural tube defects | Increased level of AFP (α-fetoprotein) (MSAFP level) |
| Ovarian tumors | Increased level of CA-125 |
| Down's Syndrome | *Decreased* level of AFP (Remember, ("Down" = Decreased") |

# Additional Topics    15

---

## CHLOASMA

This is a melasma or increased brown patches on the skin of the face or other areas (hyperpigmentation of the nipple or vagina). Chloasma is associated with *pregnancy*, *menopause*, and with *oral contraceptive use*.

---

## HIDRADENOMA

Seen in young patients (20 to 30s) from apocrine sweat glands, this is usually a solitary cyst-like mass and is NOT considered malignant.

---

## NEVUS

Pigmented nevi occur on the skin and vulva, but junctional malignant transformation is common. You may do an excisional biopsy.

---

## HEMANGIOMA

This is a congenital, small cherry angiomata, angiokeratoma, or a larger pyogenic granuloma seen during pregnancy that requires wide excision.

---

## POTTER'S SYNDROME

Renal agenesis and fetal malformations.

---

## APPENDICITIS

Patient presents with a mild fever (100.4°F), and *flank pain* or right lower quadrant abdominal pain. Also consider pyelonephritis or ovarian torsion in your differential diagnosis.

## PYELONEPHRITIS

Patient presents with a *high* fever, and *flank pain* or right lower quadrant pain.

## UTERINE INVERSION

Consider *uterine inversion* in a patient who is: *multiparous* or has a placenta in the cervical os, fresh-looking lesion, sharp increase in blood pressure *(hypertension)*, or *profuse* bleeding.

## UTERINE PROLAPSE

The uterus descends with the upper vagina. The cervix may remain *in* the vagina, protrude *past* the introitus, or descend *entirely outside* the vulva.

## DISSEMINATED INTRAVASCULAR COAGULATION (DIC)

DIC is the *consumption* of *platelets* with coagulation factor depletion, and the increase of *fibrinolysis*. It is considered a dysfunctional fibrinogen state. This condition *increases* the PT and PTT. The most common cause of DIC in pregnancy is *placental abruption*, from the release of *thromboplastin* (from the placenta into the maternal circulation) causing *consumptive coagulopathy*. Other causes include: severe preeclampsia, intrauterine fetal demise, infection or sepsis, burns, trauma, amnionic fluid embolism, and mismatched blood transfusion reactions. On histologic exam, there will be *schistocytes* on the blood smear. In treatment, you want to correct the *underlying cause*, the platelets, and give *fresh frozen plasma* (FFP) for clotting factors.

## SEIZURES

This is a neurologic disorder that may increase in occurrence during pregnancy. Treatment of seizures includes *Dilantin* and *Phenobarbital*. But, the drug of choice during pregnancy is low divided doses of *phenobarbital*—since it is less teratogenic. However, if the patient is stable with a specific regimen and she becomes pregnant, then she will usually continue with her set treatment (don't change). It is considered more harmful to the developing fetus to be hypoxic. This can occur in seizure disorders—keeping the mother seizure-free is more important. (Risk of teratogenicity is less than risks of seizures and hypoxia to the fetus.) Other anti-convulsant drugs are also used with care; these include clonazepam and carbamazepine (Tegretol). Do NOT use *valproic acid*, because of the risk of *spina bifida*, hypospadias, and craniofacial and skeletal malformations. Other problems associated with seizure medications include: fetal hydantoin syndrome, and cranio-facial anomalies, retardation, developmental delay, and neonatal withdrawal. Remember, there are teratogenic effects associated with all seizure medications.

## AUTOIMMUNE DISEASES

The following diseases will affect the maternal-fetal outcome: Rheumatoid arthritis, SLE, ITP, Grave's disease, and myasthenia gravis. The fetus is affected if an IgG antibody is produced against an organ.

## NARCOTIC DEPRESSION OF THE NEWBORN

Respiratory depression of the newborn due to excessive *narcotic* medication can be countered by *Naloxone* (Narcan). This will assist in resuscitating the neonate.

## AUTOSOMAL DOMINANT DISORDERS

There is a **50 percent** chance of the offspring expressing an abnormal gene. Some autosomal *dominant* disorders include: tuberous sclerosis, neurofibromatosis, craniofacial anomalies, adult polycystic kidney disease, and muscular dystrophy.

## AUTOSOMAL RECESSIVE DISORDERS

These disorders need *two* genes for expression of a disease. Many of the autosomal *recessive* disorders are *enzyme deficiencies*. Some examples of autosomal recessive disorders include: Tay-Sachs disease, sickle cell anemia, beta-thalassemia, and cystic fibrosis.

## SEX-LINKED DISORDERS

These disorders are linked to the X-chromosome, and are found mainly in males (females transmit to males). A couple of examples of sex-linked disorders include: Duchenne's muscular dystrophy, hemophilia, and fragile-X syndrome.

## MULTIFACTORIAL DISORDERS

Multifactorial disorders comprise the majority of *birth defects* (the genes *and* the environment play a role). Examples include: cleft lip, neural tube defects, congenital heart defects, pyloric stenosis, and anencephaly.

| Disease/Disorder | Common Treatment |
| --- | --- |
| Gonorrhea | Ceftriaxone (+ Doxycycline or Azithromycin for *C. trachomatis*) |
| Chlamydia | Azythromicin (Zithromax) or Erythromycin |
| *Trichomonas vaginalis*<br>*Gardnerella vaginitis* | Metronidazole (Flagyl) |
| *Candida albicans* | Anti-fungals (Diflucan or Fluconazole, Nystatin, Monistat cream, ketoconazole) |
| Syphilis | Penicillin G |
| Chancroid | Ceftriaxone or Erythromycin |
| *E. coli* | Cephalosporin |
| Enteric organisms | Aminoglycosides (Gentamicin) |
| Anaerobes | Clindamycin |
| Tubo-ovarian abscess | Triple-antibiotic coverage: Ampicillin, Gentamicin, and Clindamycin |
| PID | Outpatient: IM Ceftriaxone and Doxycycline orally<br>Inpatient: Cefotetan IV + Doxycycline IV or orally or Clindamycin IV + Gentamicin IV or IM |
| Urinary tract infection | Bactrim (Trimethoprim-Sulfamethoxazole) (Check sensitivity)<br>If pregnant: Ampicillin or a Cephalosporin, like Keflex or Nitrofurantoin |

| "Most Common..." | Disease/Disorder in Women |
|---|---|
| OB/Gyn admission<br>Tumor<br>Pelvic Tumor | Leiomyma |
| Ovarian Tumor<br>  Benign overian tumor<br>  Malignant ovarian tumor<br>  Cause of death in ovarian tumor | Surface epithelioma<br>  Serous Muscinous cystadenoma<br>  Serous cystadenocarcinoma<br>  Intestinal obstruction |
| *Benign* germ cell tumor | Teratoma |
| *Malignant* germ cell tumor | Dysgerminoma |
| Cancer of the Vulva | Squamous cell carcinoma |
| Vulvar tumor | Bartholin's cyst |
| Malignancy of the genital tract | Endometrial carcincoma |
| Malignant tumor | Breast tumor |
| *Benign* breast tumor | Fibroadenoma |
| *Malignant* breast tumor | Infiltrating ductal carcinoma |
| Breast disorder | Fibrocystic disease |
| Cause of bloody discharge<br>from the nipple | Intraductal lpapilloma |
| Maculinizing tumor | Arrhenoblatoma (Sertoli-Leydig tumor) |
| Endometrial hyperplasia | Cystic |
| Cause of Meig's syndrome | Fibroma |
| Cause of Vaginitis | Hemophilus vaginalis |
| Cause of urgency<br>incontinence in women | Atrophic vaginitis |
| Cause of urgency incontinence<br>in *multiparous* women | Pelvic trauma |
| Cause of stress incontinence in<br>*nulliparous* women | CNS lesion or congenital |
| Abnormality leading to<br>Urinary Tract Infection | Vesico-Ureteral reflux |

*(continued)*

| "Most Common..." | Disease/Disorder in Women |
| --- | --- |
| Cause of persistent urinary in-continence in young females | Aberrant ureter |
| Metastasis to the fetus | Melanoma |
| Abnormal presentation | Occiput Posterior |
| Cause of Anovulation | Polycystic disease |
| Cause of Infertility | Either tubal pathology or anovulation |
| Need for Hysterectomy | Myomatous uterus |
| Cause of post-partum fever | Dehydration |
| Cause of post-partum hemorrhage | Uterine atony |
| Cause of placental abruption | PIH, or Pregnancy-induced hypertension |
| Endocrine abnormality in pregnancy | Diabetes mellitus |
| Cause of Jaundice in pregnancy | Viral hepatitis |
| Complication of pregnancy | Abortion |
| Cause of abortion | Rejection of defective genetic makeup |
| Result of PROM (premature rupture of membrane) | Premature labor |
| Cause of pedal edema | Compression of IVC (inferior vena cava) |
| Injury during labor | 1. Pudendal nerve 2. Sciatic nerve |
| Complication of pitocin | Hypertonus |
| Cause of maternal death | Hemorrhage |

| Statistics in Obstetrics | In the United States |
|---|---|
| Birth rate $= \dfrac{\text{number of } live\ births}{1{,}000 \text{ population}}$ | $=$ (approximately 7 births per 1,000 population) |
| Fertility rate $= \dfrac{\text{number of } live\ births}{1{,}000 \text{ females}}$ | $=$ (approximately 680 per 1,000 females) |
| *Maternal* mortality rate $= \dfrac{\text{number of } maternal\ deaths}{100{,}000\ live\ births}$ | $=$ (about 7 mothers) die per 100,000 births) |
| (Risks: unmarried white women, increased age over 40, primigravidas, diseases, Blacks>Whites) | |
| *Infant* mortality rate $= \dfrac{\text{number of } infant\ deaths}{1{,}000\ live\ births}$ | $=$ (approx. 9/1,000) |
| (Risks: Blacks>Whites>Hispanic, and Males>Females) | |
| *Perinatal* mortality rate $= \dfrac{\text{number of } still\ births\ and\ neonatal\ deaths}{1{,}000 \text{ live births}}$ | $=$ approx. 15/1,000 |
| (Risks: Poor prenatal care and prematurity) | |

| Teratogens | Causes |
|---|---|
| Thalidomide | Phocomelia and other malformations |
| Ethanol | Fetal alcohol syndrome, prenatal growth deficiencies, craniofacial anomalies, mild to moderate mental retardation |
| Accutane (Isotretinoin) | Embryopathy; CNS, C-V, and craniofacial defects/hearing defects |
| Antianxiety drugs (Diazepam) | 1st trimester: increase in oral clefts. |
| Anticonvulsants | Given to an epileptic pregnant woman: |
| Dilantin | Fetal hydantoin syndrome; cranio-facial anomalies, retardation |

*(continued)*

| Teratogens | Causes |
|---|---|
| Valproic acid | 1–2 % risk of open spina bifida and hypospadias, cranio-facial and skeletal malformations |
| Tegretol-carbamazepine | Minor cranio-facial malformations, and developmental delay |
| Phenobarbital | Usually given in combination with other drugs; cause: neonatal withdrawal |
| Antineoplastic drugs (MTX and aminopterin), Folic acid antagonists | retardation, cranio-facial anomalies, stillbirth |
| Antibiotics | Cranial nerve damage Vestibulo-cochlear nerve, Yellow teeth |
| Coumarin | First trimester: risk for spontaneous abortion, IUGR, CNS defects, and stillbirth |
| Heparin | Does NOT cross the placenta Therefore, it can be given |
| Hormones (Progestins/Estrogens) | Pregnant woman on birth control pills: masculinization, cardiovascular and nervous system defects, sexual organ development |
| Smoking | Low birth weight and IUGR |
| Illicit drugs (cocaine) | Retardation, neurobehavioral abnormalities, and placental abruption. |
| Infectious agents (HIV, viruses, bacteria) | Infections and defects |
| Radiation | >50 cGy to fetus is teratogenic >10 cGy enough for abortion Even doses of 5 cGy may produce mutations |

## Apgar Scoring

| Signs \ Score | 0 | 1 | 2 |
|---|---|---|---|
| Cardio: Beats per minute | Absent | Slow (<100) | ≥100 |
| Respiration | Absent | Slow, Shallow Irregular | Good Crying |
| Muscle Tone | Limp | Some Flexion | Good Activity |
| Reflex Irritability | No Response | Grimace | Cry or Cough |
| Color | Pale or Blueish | Pink Body, Blue Extremities | Completely Pink |

## Bishop Pelvic Scoring
### (for elective induction of labor)

| Exam \ Score | 1 | 2 | 3 |
|---|---|---|---|
| Cervical dilatation in cm. | 1–2 | 3–4 | 5–6 |
| Cervical effacement in % | 40–50 | 60–70 | 80 |
| Station of Presentation | −1, −2 | 0 | +1, +2 |
| Consistency of Cervix | Medium | Soft | — |
| Position of Cervix | Middle | Anterior | — |

With a pelvic score of 9 or more, you may consider to safely perform an elective induction of labor.

# Index

# *Index*

The letter *f* following a page number indicates that a figure is being referenced.

Abdominal ectopic pregnancy, 52
Abortion, 41–42, 113, 130
  β-hCG, 113
  complete, 41–42, 43*f*, 44, 114
  elective, 66–67, 113, 116
  incomplete, 42, 43*f*, 44, 114
  inevitable, 41–42, 43*f*, 44, 114
  missed, 41–42, 43*f*, 44, 114
  RU 486, 116
  septic, 42, 115
  surgical methods, 115–116
  threatened, 41–42, 43*f*, 44, 114
Abruption, placental, 46–48, 47*f*, 130
Abstinence, 63
Accelerations, fetal heart rate, 20
Active phase of labor, 25
Adenomatous hyperplasia, 122
Adenomyosis, 75
Adolescent, definition of, 97
Adrenal disorders
  congenital adrenal hyperplasia, 100
  Cushing's disease, 100
  Cushing's syndrome, 100
  tumors, 101
Alcohol use, 18
Allergic vulvitis, 85
Amenorrhea, 71–72
  primary, 71–72, 103
  secondary, 72, 103–104
Amniocentesis, 110
Amnionic infusion, 67
Ampulla (fallopian tubes), 3
Anaerobes, common treatment for, 128
Analgesic and anesthetic techniques,
    111
Anatomy

fallopian tubes (oviducts), 3
  infertility and, 106–107, 106*f*
  pelvic musculature, 4-5, 5*f*
  uterus, 1–3
  vagina, 4
Androgen insensitivity syndrome, 103
Android pelvic form, 29, 30*f*
Anesthetic and analgesic techniques, 111
Anovulation, 89, 130
Antepartum, normal obstetrical care during
  common complaints
    bacterial infections, 15–16, 83–84
    Candida vulvovaginitis, 12, 85, 128
    increased urinary frequency, 13
    pica, 12
    sexually transmitted diseases. *See*
      Sexually transmitted diseases
    vaginitis, 15, 129
    viral infections, 17–18, 83
  definitions, 11
  fetal heart rate monitoring. *See* Fetal
    heart rate monitoring
  fetal surveillance
    biophysical profile, 20
    contraction stress test or oxytocin
      challenge test, 19
    fetal imaging, 24
    fetal movement counts, 18–19
    nonstress tests, 19
  genetic screening, 24
  initial prenatal evaluation, 12
  maternal complicating factors, 18
  nutritional requirements, 12
Anthropoid pelvic form, 29, 30*f*
Apgar scoring, 133
Appendicitis, 125

Molar pregnancy, 118*f*, 119
Molluscum contagiosum, 14, 83
Monozygotic twins, 55, 56*f*
Mucinous tumor, 101
Müllerian duct fusion anomalies, 89
Multifactorial disorders, 127
Multiple gestations, 55, 56*f*, 57
Myomatous uterus, 130
Myometrium, 1

Narcotic depression of the newborn, 127
Natural family planning, 63
Nervi erigentes (uterus), 3
Nevo syndrome, 55
Nevus, 125
Newborn, definition of, 97
Nonidentical twins, 56*f*, 57
Nonstress tests (NST), fetal, 19
Normal physiologic changes in pregnancy.
    *See* Pregnancy, normal physiologic
    changes in
Norplant, 66

Obstetrical care. *See* Antepartum, normal
    obstetrical care during;
    Complications of pregnancy;
    Intrapartum, normal obstetrical care
    during; Postpartum, normal obstetri-
    cal care during
Obturator internus, 4
Occiput posterior presentation, 29, 130
Occult cord prolapse, 32
Oligohydramnios, 57
Oligomenorrhea, 74, 105
Operative procedures. *See* Gynecologic and
    obstetric procedures
Outlet forceps delivery, 33
Ovarian arteries, 3
Ovarian disorders
    anovulation, 89, 130
    ectopic pregnancy, 52
    hyperthecosis, 101
    ovarian dysfunction, 104
    pelvic inflammatory disease (PID),
        89–90, 128
    polycystic disease, 89, 101, 130
    torsion, 125

tubo-ovarian abscess, 89–90, 128
tumors
    epithelial, 101, 120–121
    germ-cell, 102, 120–121
    mixed cell, 120–121
    most common, 129
    stromal, 102, 120–121
Ovarian plexus, 3
Overt cord prolapse, 32
Oviducts. *See* Fallopian tubes
Oxytocin challenge test, 19

Paget's disease, 94, 117
Pap (Papanicolaou) smear, 79–80, 110–111
Paracervical block, 111
Paracervix, 5, 6*f*
Paragard, 64
Parasitic infections, 16
Parity, definition of, 11
Peau d'orange, 93
Pedal edema, 130
Pelvic anatomy, 2*f*, 4–5, 5*f*
pelvic inlet, 29, 30*f*
Pelvic inflammatory disease (PID), 89–90,
    128
Perinatal mortality rate, 131
Perinatal timeline, 41*f*
Perineal body, 4
Periodic abstinence method, 63
Phyllodes tumor, 93
Pica, 12
PID (pelvic inflammatory disease), 89–90, 128
Piper forceps, 33
Piriformis, 4
Placenta accreta, 26
Placenta increta, 26
Placental abruption, 46–48, 47*f*, 130
Placenta percreta, 26
Placenta previa, 48, 48*f*, 49
Platypelloid pelvic form, 29, 30*f*
PMS (premenstrual syndrome), 75–76
Pneumonia, postpartum, 40
Polycystic disease, 89, 101, 130
Polyhydramnios, 57
Polymenorrhea, 74, 105
Post-coital contraception, 66
Post-dates, 11, 54
Postmenopausal bleeding, 10, 53

ISBN 0-07-038220-4

90000

9 780070 382206

LINARDAKIS:OB/GYN